Yoga Sequencing Secrets

Guiding Principles & Tools for Yoga Teachers

By Flissy Saucier

Editing by Abigail Keyes

Design by Janet Daghri, Arc Graphic Design

Cover Photo by Devon Rowland Photography

ISBN: Amazon Print on Demand Paperback: 978-1-7342939-0-6

©2019 Flissy Saucier
All Rights Reserved

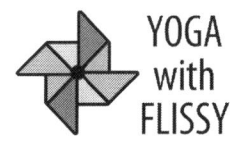

YOGA with FLISSY

yogawithflissy.com

YOGA with FLISSY

yogawithflissy.com

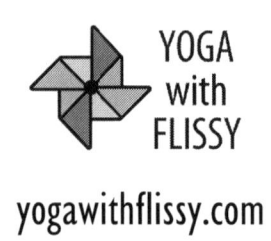

Contents

Introduction — 1
    Why Sequencing Matters — 1
    For Yoga Teachers — 1
    My Perspective — 1
    My Goals for You — 2

Chapter 1: Yoga Sequencing Principles — 3
    Ask Yourself: What is Your BIG WHY? — 3
    Warm Up, Middle, Cool Down — 4
    Be Aware of Planes — 4
    Use Proper Preparation and Compensation — 5
    Move from Simple to Complex — 6
    Check Your Symmetry — 6
    Consider the Risks — 6
    Use Variations — 7
    Understand the Benefits of Yoga Sequencing Principles — 7

Chapter 2: Consider the Context — 9
    Who are you teaching? — 9
    When are you teaching? — 10
    Where are you teaching? — 10
    What are you teaching? — 10

Chapter 3: Yoga Sequencing Pitfalls — 13
    Static Postures First — 13
    Too Complicated Too Early — 13
    Poor Preparation and/or Compensation — 13
    Too Many Postures — 14
    Yoga Choreography — 14
    Ego Driven — 14

Chapter 4: The Magical Worksheet — 17
    1. What is the intention? — 17

2. What are the core postures?	18
3. What's the context?	18
4. Student demographics and level of experience	18
5. What do your students WANT?	18
6. What are the potential risks and things to avoid?	18
7. What else might you take into consideration?	18
Draft Your Sequence	19
Magical Worksheet Sample Sequence	20
Backbend Slow Flow Practice from Magical Worksheet	21

Chapter 5: The Magical Outline — 23

Centering	23
Opening Sequence	24
Spine	24
Hips & Legs	24
Featured Topic	24
Seated and Supine	24
Finishing Sequence	25
Relaxation and Meditation	25
Adapting for Other Styles	25
Magical Outline Sample Sequence	26

Chapter 6: Yoga Court — 27

Chapter 7: Applications — 29

Long Term Planning	29
Easily Adjust Existing Material	29
Keep Up With Ongoing Teaching Demands	29
Build Your Collection	29

Chapter 8: Working in Specific Contexts — 31

Planning for Mixed Levels	31
Sequencing for Beginner Students	31
One-on-One	32
Restorative/Yin	32
Vinyasa/Flow	32
Other Traditions	32
Final Thoughts	32

Chapter 9: Sample Sequences — 33

1: A Sequence to Address Poor Posture	34
2: A Sequence to Address Chronic Stress	35
3: A Sequence to Address Dysfunctional Breathing Patterns	36

4: A Sequence to Build up to a Pinnacle Posture	37
5: A Sequence to Explore a Posture in Different Ways	43
6: A Sequence to Explore a Direction of Movement	44
7: A Sequence to Explore a Joint	45
8: Potpourri Practice	46
Same Sequence, Different Contexts	48

Conclusion — 49

Appendix — 51

Blank Worksheets	52
Yoga Sequence Worksheet	53
Yoga Sequence Outline	54
Yoga Court Checklist	55

Further Reading — 56

Introduction

Why Sequencing Matters

Many people who are unfamiliar with or perhaps new to yoga might look at asana as disconnected postures created for a specific physical benefit in the body. For example, someone might ask a yoga teacher, "What pose should I do for my back pain?" or look in a book for postures that might help alleviate shoulder discomfort.

But if you're reading this book, you probably understand that yoga postures are not a quick fix for what ails you. You can't say "Do three cobras and call me next week!" We feel the benefits of yoga when we create and practice longer sequences of postures crafted for a specific purpose or benefit. And, of course, the real power of yoga comes with consistent practice over a long period of time. That person with the low back pain isn't going to find relief in random postures done whenever they feel like doing them.

The benefits, risks, and applications of postures depend on the relationship to what comes before and after in a practice, as well as the practitioner themselves. With all that in mind (and more), I've written this book to help practitioners and instructors craft effective, safe, and thoughtful yoga sequences for themselves and their students. Whether you're a student of yoga looking to deepen your practice or a teacher who wants to create more beneficial classes, this book will help you understand how to craft sequences that consider a range of factors including the practitioner/student, the time of day, experience levels, exploring specific range of movements, and other elements of modern life such as poor posture.

For Yoga Teachers

I have found that most yoga teacher trainings don't include in-depth information about sequencing postures, and that it's difficult to find reliable resources on the topic. To help fill that gap, I'm here to support yoga teachers by sharing my expertise. I hope that by following the principles outlined in this book, teachers can improve the quality of their group classes and make them safer and more satisfying for practitioners. If you are a teacher, this is good for your students, because they will feel great and keep coming back to your class. It's good for you, because you will feel confident about teaching quality content and you will build your clientele because of your expertise. It's good for the entire profession, because when we are more knowledgeable as a whole, the public more highly values our work.

In addition to sharing my tips for sequencing, this book will help you save time as you prepare your classes. I consistently hear yoga teachers express how stressful and time consuming lesson planning can be. This book will demystify the process and reduce burnout by giving you simple step-by-step approaches to building practices. The more you use these tools and methods, the faster you'll be able to whip up a practice that you can use in multiple contexts—even in less than 30 minutes!

My Perspective

I've based this book on twenty years of yoga practice and ten years experience teaching Viniyoga, vinyasa, hatha, and yin yoga to a wide variety of individuals in a wide variety of contexts. My most influential teachers have all come from the Krishnamacharya lineage, which teaches that yoga is to be adapted to the individual, a concept that often gets lost in group classes or buried in dogma when particular styles are established. What do I mean by that? When yoga teachers guide group classes, they generally do their best to give instructions that will apply to the majority of the group. That, in itself, is generally a good approach. The problem is that teachers accept specific instructions like "turn in your back leg exactly 45 degrees" in *trikonasana* (triangle) or sequencing patterns like "always do *matsyasana* (fish) immediately after *sarvangasana* (shoulderstand)," repeating these cues to their own students as fixed truths without considering why those conventions exist or the value of deviating from those conventions when working with an individual or specific population.

If we take a step back and look at the big picture of the legacy of Krishnamacharya, we can see the personalization of yoga practice through B. K. S. Iyengar, Patthabhi Jois, T. K. V. Desikachar, Indra Devi, and many others who were all students of Krishnamacharya, and yet have radically different approaches to teaching based on what he taught them and what they understood as the most valuable information. Teachers today can learn from them that the tradition of yoga is not only about delivering specific postures and information, but practicing critical thinking and care for students as unique individuals.

My two main teachers are Gary Kraftsow and Erich Schiffmann; while they're both students of Desikachar, they are very different from one another. Gary Kraftsow (and Viniyoga in general) places a significant emphasis on the art and science of sequencing, which is the foundation of what I've included in this book. Erich Schiffmann, on the other hand, teaches that there is inherent wisdom and potential for freedom within us all, so a big part of yoga is about developing self-trust and self-expression, then employing that refined power of intuition to create enjoyable, nourishing yoga practices.

In addition to my extensive yoga experience, I am also a personal trainer and professional dancer, and my fitness background further informs how I develop yoga sequences. My diverse training has taught me that at the heart of transmitting yoga practice is the service of helping people simply feel better in their body, mind, and spirit, and there are many valid approaches to that end.

My Goals for You

My number one goal as a teacher is to empower people to do their own practice. I do this through teaching traditional yoga techniques, critical thinking, and self-trust. You will find the same anti-dogmatic approach to crafting yoga sequences, based on flexible guiding principles. Even if your background in yoga is different from mine (which it nearly certainly is!), you will be able to apply the principles and approaches to suit your own needs. I believe that everyone deserves an effective and enjoyable movement practice.

I hope that this book will provide you with tools and ideas to bring into your own practice and teaching, and inspire you to think creatively about how you craft meaningful practices for yourself and your students.

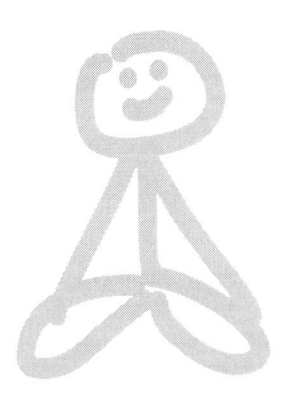

Yoga Sequencing Principles

In this chapter, I introduce the main principles that I use to create sound and organized yoga sequences. I've included some activities for you to complete to help you integrate these principles into your sequencing planning.

Ask Yourself: What is Your BIG WHY?

Before you even think about putting together a yoga sequence, take some time to **identify and connect with your BIG WHY**. Your BIG WHY answers the questions: "Why do I practice yoga?" And if you're a teacher, it also answers the question, "Why do I teach yoga?" Having answers to those questions gives context to your practice and teaching, and will inspire you to create meaningful practices. Once you have identified your BIG WHY, your yoga sequence will then answer the question: "How am I going to practice or teach that today?" When you have a purpose to your teaching and communicate your objectives to your students, you are better able to motivate them to learn and engage more fully in the practice.

Suggested Exercise:

Your BIG WHY
Journal: What is your BIG WHY?
How might you express your BIG WHY through a yoga practice?

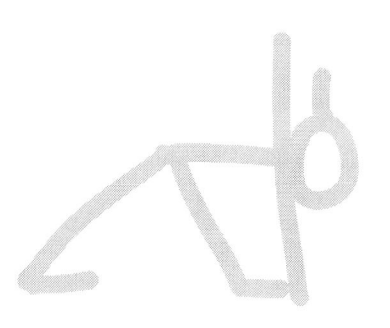

Start with a Simple Intention

An **intention** gives your practice purpose and direction; it can be physical, energetic, or thematic. A physical intention could relate to a specific body part, a direction of movement, or posture family; it might also work towards a pinnacle posture. The physical practice of doing yoga can also have powerful effects on the nervous system, so you might want to structure a practice to be energizing or calming. A thematic intention can be used to deliver a philosophical message or tell a story through the postures and arc of the sequence. Yoga asana practice can also be used as preparation for deeper work with *pranayama* and meditation, and in this case, the sequence would be in the service of whatever specific *pranayama*, *kriya*, *mantra*, or meditation practice that will follow.

Use the suggested exercise below to clarify and define your intentions before your next practice.

> **Suggested Exercise:**
>
> # Find your intention
>
> **Journal: Ask yourself the following questions before sequencing your next practice or class.**
>
> 1. Why are you doing this particular practice?
> 2. What do you want your students to learn?
> 3. What is the end result you'd like to achieve?

Apply Anatomy Knowledge

Even though yoga is far more than a fitness practice, most yoga practices incorporate movement, so yoga teachers are expected to **understand general fitness principles of musculoskeletal anatomy, kinesiology, and biomechanics**. Remember that you will be guiding other people's bodies into various movements and positions that may be unfamiliar to them.

Be sure you know the major muscles, bones, and joints of the body, as well as their function, how they move, and the typical range of motion to expect from the major joints. You should also be able to apply this textbook information to yoga practice and identify what joints and muscles are involved in various yoga postures and transitions between them.

Warm Up, Middle, Cool Down

Yoga sequences should follow the general and logical arc of a typical physical fitness session, including **a warm up** to prepare the body for movement; **a middle**, in which the practitioner does the bulk of the exercising and/or challenging movement; and **a cool down** to integrate the benefits of the practice and reduce the heart rate if the practice was rigorous.

A yoga **warm up** will fulfill the standard fitness purpose of increasing circulation, lubricating joints, and creating warmth in muscles; it will also establish the mind-body connection, an essential yoga practice foundation. In some approaches to yoga, the warm up also sets the relationship between breath and movement. In many of the sequences that I teach, the warm up postures primarily address the points of stress, explore range of motion in the joints used in the core postures, warm up the surrounding muscles, and develop the mind-body connection to coordinate the movement. After a few minutes of centering, which might include a short meditation or focus on breathing technique, the warm up sequence should include a few simple dynamic movements. A typical warm up for an hour or 90-minute long class should take about five to seven minutes. Take a look at my sample sequences in Chapter 9 for examples of yoga warm ups.

After the introductory breathing and warm-up postures, the practice proceeds to the **middle**, including the main postures. The bulk of your yoga practice should focus on the heart of your intention, whether it be mind-body connection, strength, endurance, flexibility, or anything else you choose to focus on for that practice. The middle of your practice depends entirely on your intention as well as the style of yoga you're teaching. For example, the middle portion of a a Vinyasa or flow style class focuses on standing postures and may include moving through strenuous single leg balance or arm balance postures. In contrast, when I teach a restorative practice, I'll often include some dynamic movement in the warm up, then the static postures are all in the middle section. If the intention is to work towards a pinnacle posture, the sequence should begin with simpler postures that build to one challenging posture, followed by some gentler counterposes. Or, if the intention is to teach a concept, the middle might consist of a few mini-sequences that relate directly to that concept.

Finally, your practice should end with a **cool down**. In general fitness contexts, the cool down will ease the heart rate back to a resting rhythm and sometimes include stretching. In a yoga practice, this ending sequence also activates the parasympathetic nervous system, which is a division of the central nervous system responsible for digestion, slowing the heart rate, and relaxing the muscles while the body is at rest. Activating the parasympathetic nervous system helps the practitioner reduce the symptoms of stress and feel more relaxed. The cool down also allows time and space for the practitioner to integrate the benefits of the practice. Depending on the style of class, a sequence of finishing postures could be about five to ten minutes followed by a few minutes or longer to rest in *savasana* (corpse pose).

Be Aware of Planes

If you're a fitness professional, you're probably familiar with the anatomical planes of the body: coronal, sagittal, and transverse. But in this book, I'll use the term "planes" to refer to the practitioner's relationship to the ground:

Inversions and Arm Balances

Inversions—a special category of postures where the head is lower than the heart, such as *sirsasana* (headstand)—and many arm balances require special preparation and strength conditioning. Depending on the orientation, they may require a different point of entry such as standing for *adho mukha vrksasana* (handstand) or supine for *sarvangasana*. Although *adho mukha svanasana* (downward facing dog) is technically an inversion, it is a useful transition posture because the knees can come down to the floor to move into and out of *balasana* (child's pose) or a seated position, or the feet can walk into and out of *uttanasana* (standing forward bend). *Cakravakasana* (hands and knees to child's pose) and *vajrasana* (standing on knees to child's pose) are Viniyoga favorites for moving between planes because they are simple forward bends that also serve as counterposes.

kneeling, standing, prone (lying on the belly), supine (lying on the back), seated, and inverted. Your sequencing should **consider how you transition between one plane to another**, as well as how often. For example, if you're moving up and down from the floor, it is best to transition through kneeling, as going from standing to lying down (or vice versa) can create unnecessary stress on the body. In particular, moving from supine, as in *dwi pada pittham* (bridge), immediately to standing, in *tadasana* (mountain), can cause a drop in blood pressure and lead to dizziness, light-headedness, or fainting. Similarly, lying down on your back in *savasana* immediately after a strenuous sequence of standing postures, can cause unnecessary strain to your nervous and pulmonary system and make it difficult to relax, which is the exact opposite of why we do *savasana*.

Organize your sequence so that you or your students practice a group of postures in one plane before going to the next. This sequence will be less strenuous than a practice that has many transitions up and down from the ground. An elegant yoga sequence will flow seamlessly from one plane to the next without additional strain or discomfort to the practitioner. You can make your practices simpler and safer by minimizing transitions between planes.

Use Proper Preparation and Compensation

One of the most important principles for reducing risk of injury and minimizing any stressful side effects of more intense yoga postures is integrating proper **preparation and compensation** into your sequencing. Preparation is the use of simpler postures in a logical sequence to ready the body for what follows. Compensation includes the use of counterposes, which are generally simpler postures that move in the opposite direction from the core posture. More importantly, compensation is the use of postures that systematically address the areas of body that are under stress in the core posture. Use of proper preparation and compensation is particularly important when working on complex postures—such as *janu sirsasana parivrtti* (revolved head to knee)—which includes a bind, an asymmetrical foundation, and a combination of forward bending and twisting. Use preparation postures that incorporate each of these main attributes before combining them all at once in the core posture. Then, follow up with compensation postures that address the areas of stress, which in this case are the sacroiliac joint, low back, and shoulders. Remember that preparation and compensation postures should be simpler and gentler than the core posture.

Simple forward bends are essential compensation as transition between directions of movement. When you are teaching a class with backbends, twists, and lateral bends, make sure you plan a simple forward bend to transition to another direction. Simple forward bends stretch the muscles around the low back and restore the spine to a neutral alignment before moving on to the next postures. They also reduce the risk of muscle spasms or excessive compression to the intervertebral discs. When you are practicing an extreme range of movement—particularly with backbends as in *ustrasana* (camel)—choose simple forward bends like *balasana* or *apanasana* (supine knees to chest) instead of intense ones like *pascimatanasana* (seated forward bend), which could cause undue strain. That said, it is fine to add longer or more intense forward bends later in the practice as general compensation for all the backbending that preceded.

In addition, consider adding resting postures as compensation between more rigorous sequences. Neutral positions such as *savasana*, *apanasana*, *balasana*, *sukhasana* (easy seated position), and *tadasana* give practitioners a chance to integrate whatever they did prior and make space for them to proceed to the next posture mindfully.

Overall, the whole sequence should be balanced, with a logical progression of building up and winding down across the the entirety of the practice. For an example of proper preparation and compensation, look at A Sequence to Build Up to a Pinnacle Posture in Chapter 9.

Move from Simple to Complex

Just as we need to understand arithmetic before we can do algebra, your yoga sequences should introduce simple concepts and postures before moving on to more complex ones. No matter how advanced your students, make sure the beginning of your sequences include fundamental actions of postures and transitions. This progression will help your students ease into their practice so they can evaluate how their body is feeling. With that mindful awareness, they'll be able to move safely and and freely. They'll also be able to apply foundational skills more effectively to challenging postures, and use these skills in combination with others in the future. There are two ways we can move from simple to complex: **general to subtle** and **gentle to strong**.

A sequence that progresses from **general to subtle** will begin with big, whole body movements and then progress to refined movements that are specific to individual joints or body parts. For example, a practice focused on flexion and extension of the spine might begin with *uttanasana* then proceed to *parsvottanasana* (single leg forward bend), which introduces an asymmetrical element. It might also include simple backbends like *virabhadrasana* (warrior I), which has a larger, unfixed range of motion followed later by *bhujangasana* (cobra), which more specifically works the spinal extensors. The end of the practice may include *mahamudra* (great seal), an extension posture where the practitioner can subtly adjust the spinal curves while staying in the posture. You can also apply this approach to help students understand the big picture of a posture or transition, from which they can refine their understanding and execution, by giving more details each time you repeat a posture in class.

Working **gentle to strong** will begin with postures requiring less muscular effort and progress to postures and/or transitions that are more strenuous or difficult. If you wish to move from gentle to strong, you should consider your yoga planes. Generally speaking, the progression of planes from most gentle to most strenuous is: supine, kneeling, standing, seated, inverted. While seated postures don't require as much muscular effort as some standing postures (particularly standing balance postures), the pelvis is fixed and therefore more strain can be transferred to the low back. Postures with a broad foundation—like standing postures with a wide stance—are more gentle than unstable postures, so simple standing postures with both feet grounded should precede single-leg balances.

When considering whether your elements are gentle or strong, you should identify whether a pose is **free or fixed**; free or open postures are more gentle than fixed ones. In free postures, the joints are uninhibited, as in *salabhasana* (locust), where the torso, arms, and legs may lift off the floor to any degree and in any position. Fixed postures incorporate binds or other positions where limbs might be used as levers. *Dhanurasana* (bow) is more strenuous than *salabhasana* because the hands grip the ankles, creating a fixed frame and leverage for the backbend.

You'll also want to consider whether your postures are **weight bearing or non-weight bearing**. Weight bearing postures are stronger than non-weight bearing ones. Even though the body might be in the same anatomical shape in different postures, the body might be bearing weight very differently in each. For example, in both *virabhadrasana* and *adho mukha svanasana*, the shoulders are in flexion when the arms are overhead, but in *adho mukha svanasana* the arms and shoulders are weight bearing while in *virabhadrasana* they are not. If you are planning a sequence to progressively work the shoulders more strongly, place *virabhadrasana* earlier in the sequence to prepare the shoulders for that additional work.

When moving from gentle to strong, also consider whether your postures are **static or dynamic**. Generally speaking, doing a posture dynamically is more gentle than holding it statically. For example, moving in and out of *utkatasana* (chair) from standing is less strenuous than staying for the equal number of breaths because it requires more endurance and strength to hold the half-squat position. That being said, in a restorative or yin style practice, a seated posture may be completely supported by props and in that case, long holds can be the gentler approach.

Check Your Symmetry

In addition to planning adequate preparation and compensation, **check the use of asymmetrical postures** in your practice. Too many asymmetrical postures in a row can cause unnecessary strain to the sacroiliac joint. However, asymmetrical postures can also help address muscular imbalance and prepare for symmetrical postures by working each side separately (which is often less strenuous than recruiting the whole body). Therefore, a balanced use of symmetrical and asymmetrical postures is often the most beneficial.

Consider the Risks

If you're reading this book, you understand that yoga can be incredibly beneficial to the mind and body. But there are inherent **physiological and energetic risks** in any yoga practice, depending on the practitioner, postures, and individual needs of the student.

Many yoga postures or transitions can cause physical harm to to the joints, muscles, and connective tissues of the body if a practitioner isn't properly warmed up, prepared, or strong enough. A practitioner could injure themselves in a yoga practice through repetition of certain postures, going into a posture that is beyond their range of motion, or doing postures that are contraindicated for their specific demographic or prior conditions. You must consider these factors when planning your yoga sequences. For example, if you teach vinyasa classes, the constant use of transitioning through *caturanga dandasana* (low plank) in sun salutations may cause repetitive use injuries to the wrists, elbows, or shoulders.

Many people come to yoga with existing conditions such as osteoporosis. For those people, forward bends or other movements may be contraindicated entirely, or may require specific preparation or adaptations for them to practice them safely. Make sure your sequence includes adequate preparation, and make sure to vary your sequencing over the long term to reduce the risk of injuries or strain due to overuse.

And, as we explored earlier, complex variations of postures tend to be riskier than simpler ones for a variety of reasons: leverage created by binds, straining to achieve a particular shape, or imbalances becoming injuries when a body is pushed to its limits. I have known several practitioners injure their groins, hamstrings, or shoulders attempting full *svarga dvijasana* (bird of paradise), a posture that challenges a practitioner's range of motion, balance, and arm bind under the thigh. Others have torn their hamstrings by attempting yoga tricks like *hanumanasana* (splits) without adequate warm up.

In addition to strains and tears, another potential risk is falling. While seniors are often at a higher risk of falling than other populations, it is important to consider this risk in other contexts as practitioners of all ages and experience may topple out of balance postures and inversions. Falling becomes even more of a concern in a crowded studio, where one person losing their balance could injure other practitioners. When you incorporate postures that challenge balance, remember to include postures that train strength, core stability, and awareness before introducing your main balance postures. Consider if you can use props for support, such as walls or sturdy chairs. If you're including balances or inversions, make sure you plan adequate time to support everyone's individual needs; you might also have small groups or individuals go one at a time if you feel they need a spotter or simply more space to work.

Yoga postures and breathing exercises also can have powerful energetic effects that affect blood pressure and/or the nervous system and therefore may not be appropriate for all populations. As mentioned previously, sequences that have many transitions from standing to seated or supine can disrupt blood pressure and cause people to be light-headed or dizzy. Your sequence might also have unintended psychosomatic effects. For example, an energizing practice full of backbends, followed by a stimulating *pranayama* practice, may cause someone who already has anxiety to have a full blown panic attack. If you choose to do practices that may stress the nervous system, makes sure you also plan time for finishing postures to bring the body back into balance as well as several minutes to rest in *savasana* at the end.

Use Variations

You can maximize the benefit (and minimize the risk) of postures by using **variations** and props such as straps, blocks, blankets, and bolsters. A strap in *supta padangusthasana* (hand to big toe) can help extend reach, and a block under the hand in *ardha chandrasana* (half moon) can bring the floor closer, reducing the potential for injury or strain. You can also vary postures by changing arm positions, bending the knees, or decreasing the load, which will make postures more accessible or gentle. These modifications can also help prepare the muscles and joints for more strenuous work.

As a yoga teacher, it is your responsibility to be aware of the general contraindications and risk for injury associated with the positions and movements used in yoga practice. These considerations are not to scare you off from ever attempting strenuous, difficult, or risky positions or transitions; just about everything we do in our daily life has some inherent risk. But if you use intelligent sequencing, use of props and variations, you and your students will benefit from a yoga practice while reducing potential ill effects. And, many of the risks associated with particular postures can be minimized by proper preparation and compensation, which is why having a fundamental understanding of anatomy and biomechanics is so essential for creating safe yoga sequences. Most importantly, the postures and transitions you choose should be based on the population and context you are working with.

Understand the Benefits of Yoga Sequencing Principles

Without intentional sequencing, yoga postures are puzzle pieces scattered all over a table, and when put in order, through a logical sequence, they create a pleasing picture that makes sense. When you take the time to **understand the sequencing principles** and connect them to the practices you already do, you will better understand individual yoga postures and how to use them for the best benefit. You'll also be able to develop safer yoga practices that will help you and your students more effectively learn the material you are teaching and consistently feel better at the end of class.

Suggested Exercise:

Evaluate an existing sequence

Look at one of your yoga lesson plans (or make a new one) and see how it measures up to the sequencing principles. What looks strong about your sequence? How might you change it to align more strongly with the sequencing principles?

Consider the Context

One of the best things about yoga is that the teachings are universal and available to all who are interested. That said, it can be challenging to deliver that promise, because not all yoga practices are appropriate for all people all of the time. It takes some preparation to ensure that your practices are accessible and beneficial to the people you are working with. While my yoga sequencing principles give you the general foundation for a practice, you'll also need to consider the context in which you'll use the practice. Doing so will help you identify the specific postures and variations you'll choose, as well as how you'll apply them. You'll also be able to create yoga sequences that fit the exact time, population and location in which you're teaching them.

Who are you teaching?

Within the Krishnamacharya lineage, as well as in other yoga traditions, teachings were usually transmitted from teacher to student one-on-one and specifically tailored to suit the student's needs. Taking your student into consideration when you plan a sequence both honors the tradition of yoga and ensures that you'll deliver a practice that is as safe and beneficial as possible. When working with groups of students, consider the general setting of the class and give your best estimate of what your students may need based on the overall demographic of the group. You should also consider your students' prior yoga experience, general level of fitness and mobility, their occupation and lifestyle, as well as their age.

When you know your students have little experience with yoga and/or other movement or fitness practices, it's best to start with the simplest concepts, postures, and transitions. Then you can evaluate what they are able to do before getting into complex or strenuous postures. And even though your students might already exercise regularly, that doesn't necessarily mean that they are proficient at yoga. Preparing sequences for newer students can often be challenging, because they won't know how to adapt postures to suit their own needs or rest as needed without your assistance or direction. Make sure you are prepared to teach modifications and other variations; you'll not only teach a safer class, but your students will also feel that they are benefitting from the practice even if they are unable to do more complex versions of postures.

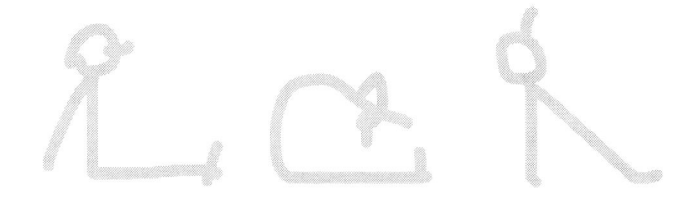

Even if you don't know the details about your individual students, you might be able to get a general idea of the demographic based on when and where you are teaching. For example, you may teach at a fitness club used by endurance athletes who take yoga classes on their rest days from training. In this case, you might want to craft a sequence designed to improve muscle recovery. Or, you may teach a class attended by many young parents right after dropping their children off at school in the morning, so you might plan an energizing sequence to start their day. If you teach a lunchtime class in a corporate environment, your students might need more stress management or compensation for sitting.

You'll certainly want to consider your students' age as well. While age is not necessarily an indicator of physical ability, generally speaking, older folks in particular can benefit from strength training and balance, though they may have limited mobility or strength to start with as both of these qualities naturally deteriorate with age. You might also want to consider props and other elements to help less mobile older students get the most out of the practice without strain or risk of injury.

Some classes will have a very diverse demographic. In these cases, identify the foundation of your sequence, and look for places where your students needs and interests intersect. As you plan, keep in mind how you can make everyone feel included and able to participate fully.

When are you teaching?

It might not be obvious, but when you teach your class is just as important as who is in your class. As I've mentioned before, yoga postures can have a powerful effect on the nervous system. The Sanskrit terminology for these effects are *langhana* (relaxing, nourishing), *samana* (balanced), and *brmhana* (energizing). Though the nuances of these energetic effects can be quite complex, a good general guideline is that morning is best for *brmhana* or energizing practices, and evening is best for *langhana* or relaxing practices.

With this in mind, you probably won't want to put relaxing postures together for a class at 6:30am full of students who will go to a corporate office afterwards. And if you're teaching a class at 8:00pm, you probably don't want to use a lot of energizing postures that might prevent your students from falling asleep when they get home.

What does this mean for choices of yoga postures? Energizing postures include backbends, lateral bends, more repetition or flow, and a generally more strenuous practice. Relaxing postures include twists and forward bends, staying in a posture longer, and a generally more gentle practice. It's perfectly fine to include backbends or stimulating postures in the evening, just make sure to balance the practice with adequate time to relax through more gentle postures towards the end. It's also not wrong to include relaxing postures in an early morning practice, as long as they are balanced with some dynamic movement and you provide a transition to being awake and alert, perhaps through some seated *pranayama* or meditation.

In addition to the time of the day, also take into consideration what else might be happening in your students' day. Are they rushing to class directly to or from work? Is class the first thing they do to start off a relaxing weekend day? Thinking about how yoga practice fits into your students' routine will inform which postures you choose as well as the intensity of the practice.

Where are you teaching?

The physical environment where you teach—the location, length of the class, and availability of props—may also influence the postures you choose. A noisy gym and a quiet yoga studio are very different spaces, with different props available. A yoga studio will likely have props specific to yoga, you have a lot more options for incorporating variations on postures. It's also more likely to be quiet and have fewer distractions than other locations.

Let's look at the challenges presented by teaching yoga in a gym environment. Because the sound of music or weights dropping can be distracting, people often need a little longer to focus on being in class, and they might benefit from a longer warm up. The noise might also distract students from relaxing at the end of class, so you might use a sequence of several seated and supine postures to keep people focused on the experience of the practice rather than staying in just one or two, which might allow students' minds to be distracted by outside noise.

Other situations pose their own challenges. If you are using a community space that has only chairs and no mats, you may have to come up with specific postures, variations, and transitions based on what is available. If you are working one-on-one with a student, you may be teaching them in their own home with all the obstacles and distractions that go along with that, so you may create a shorter sequence they can do on their own when they have limited time. If you know the space in advance, with a little creativity, you can plan a practice that fulfills your intention and meets your students needs, even if it seems less than ideal for whatever reason.

In addition to the physical space, you might also have to adapt your practice to fit a time constraint or fill more time than what you're used to teaching. For example, if you're crafting a 30-minute lunch break practice you can pare down your sequence to only essential postures. If you're teaching a longer workshop, you can fill out that 30-minute practice with more rest time and complimentary postures.

What are you teaching?

The final piece to consider is efficiency of the sequence. Once you have planned your sequence, look back and see if you have made the best choices by evaluating your sequence based on the principles and considerations discussed. Is there anything extra that can be cut out or transitions that can be made more elegant by grouping similar postures together? It is also useful to try out your sequence and see how it feels in your own body. Practicing your sequences will help you learn what makes a sequence have a good flow and how it feels to implement the principles and considerations in a practice. When you practice your sequence to look for a sense of flow, keep in mind the context in which you plan to use the sequence.

Remember that everyone is unique and what works for you might not work for your students. If you have any postures or transitions that seem like they could be tricky for certain populations, note how you might teach them and what options to offer to set your students up for success. Elegance and flow are subjective and are the artistic elements that balance the more objective sequencing principles and will evolve with practice. Explore these more subtle aspects of sequencing and develop your unique voice as a teacher by journalling about how practices feel and how they are received by your students.

Suggested Exercise:
Clarify your context
Journal: Answer the following questions.
1. Who are you teaching?
2. When are you teaching?
3. Where are you teaching?
4. How might you best serve your clientele in these various contexts?

Yoga Sequencing Pitfalls

Before we get into how to apply the principles to create effective yoga sequences, let's take a look at some of the common sequencing pitfalls. Some of these pitfalls are intrinsic to particular styles or schools of yoga, and so we'll simply explore why some sequencing choices might be problematic. Then we'll dig into how to make safer and more informed choices. If you realize that you have made these mistakes, don't be discouraged! When you've finished reading this section, you'll be more empowered to avoid these pitfalls as you plan your next practice.

Static Postures First

In general, you want to avoid doing static postures at the beginning of your practice. Without a proper warm up, they can be difficult and cause muscle cramping. They also make the practitioner more vulnerable to tears and strains, because the muscles lack the elasticity they gain from dynamic movement. Teachers sometimes place seated postures like *pascimatanasana* or *sukhasana parivrtti* (seated twist) at the beginning of class because it seems intuitive: after all, you're probably already sitting. However, static seated postures like these are particularly problematic because the pelvis is fixed and therefore can transfer unnecessary stress to the low back and sacroiliac joint.

A better choice: Include some kind of movement at the beginning of your practice. I love starting with cat/cow or *cakravakasana*, because it introduces gentle flexion and extension of the spine through dynamic movement.

Too Complicated Too Early

Teachers under pressure to get the most out of an hour long class or serve students who crave sweaty, strenuous practices sometimes jump right into stringing postures together in complicated flows. As in the case of doing static postures first, complicated postures and transitions at the beginning of practice also put participants at risk of injury due to a lack of warm up. In addition, when teaching a class, delivering too much information at once can be overwhelming and difficult for students to process. If a student gets frustrated right off the bat, it is challenging to get their attention and good spirits back for the remainder of the practice.

A better choice: Keep the beginning of your sequence simple, then build to more complex or demanding postures as the practice progresses.

Poor Preparation and/or Compensation

Inadequate preparation, including lack of warm up or lack of awareness of the body's limitations, can lead to higher risk of injury. It is common for teachers or practitioners to go directly from one direction of movement or concept to something completely different without compensation or transition. Generally, this is due to a lack of understanding about sequencing and how the relationship between yoga postures in a sequence is just as important as the individual postures themselves. Arbitrarily moving from one posture to the next can create unresolved residual stress from the previous posture and be generally jarring to the flow of the practice.

Many people misunderstand counterposes as postures that are "opposite" to others, but the reality is more nuanced. A counterpose that is too strenuous—for example, going from *urdhva dhanurasana* (upward facing bow) directly to *pascimatanasana*—can cause muscle spasms or excessive disc compression in the spine. In vinyasa or flow practices, it is common for there to be a lack of adequate cool down, which stresses the nervous system and makes it hard for students to rest in *savasana*. Going directly from standing to supine also is risky for blood pressure regulation.

A better choice: Look carefully at the postures in your practice. If you have a demanding posture or sequence planned, it should include a logical progression building up to the most challenging part. If you have a series of demanding postures, incorporate simple forward bends in between each. Make sure that the final sequences in your practice compensate for the stress accumulated in the practice, paying special attention to any areas in the body that may have been susceptible to increased risk.

Too Many Postures

It is easy as a teacher to want to cram in as much information as possible; however, if a practice has too many postures, students will not have adequate time to explore the mind-body connection in each posture or integrate understanding of what they are doing. A long sequence of postures presented in a rush can cause students to scramble to keep up and unintentionally strain a muscle or stress a joint in the process. If a practice has too many postures that are randomly incorporated, it will feel unfocused or unbalanced.

A better choice: Simplify your practice by picking two or three postures that best support the ideas or skills you want to teach, then build your sequence around those few postures. A general guideline for a 60-minute asana practice is about 12-20 postures. If it is a restorative or yin practice with longer holds, or if you are including significant time in *savasana*, *pranayama*, or meditation, your practice will have fewer postures.

Yoga Choreography

Yoga is in the service of developing a better relationship between mind and body and includes inner practices of *pranayama*, meditation, and reflection on philosophical teachings. Without these inner practices, yoga postures are randomly practiced together with no other context, and they can be reduced to fancy calisthenics. Even when yoga teachers understand and place value on the deeper teachings of yoga, if they overemphasize the postural practice, their class risks turning into what I call "yoga choreography." The practice becomes a string of physical movements that practitioners execute exactly as directed, more like an aerobics class than a tradition based in mindfulness and mind-body awareness.

How does this happen if yoga teachers know that the practice is more than just postures? Yoga teachers often feel immense pressure to create novel, unconventional classes, particularly ones with tricky transitions to give students a physical workout. That's not to say that challenging practices are always bad! But if you're trying to complicate your practice in order to create something "new," consider how this might not be to the best benefit of your students.

A better choice: Consider how a strenuous practice can be in service of a deeper message. Plan how to share deeper layers of yoga teaching in class or explain the benefit of doing a strenuous or complex physical practice. Many people are drawn to sweaty flow practices, and so if you choose to practice or teach this kind of practice, proper compensation is especially important to bring the body and nervous system back into balance before proceeding with the rest of your day.

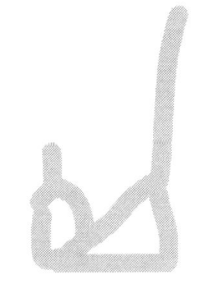

Ego Driven

An extreme example of ego driven sequences are yoga classes that are based on showing off what a teacher can do rather than teaching content relevant to their students. Yoga teachers often create lesson plans for their students strictly based on their own practice. While this is a fine place to start, we teachers are in service of our students. Due to your unique anatomical structure, level of fitness, lifestyle, and preferences, you may love postures and approaches that may be impossible for your students. Remember that what feels great in your body might be inappropriate, or even harmful for others.

Successful instructors have an objective and almost analytical understanding of yoga practice, including the purpose of individual postures and their relationship to one another. If you are only ever doing practices intuitively, it is likely you have blind spots such as postures or directions of movement that you avoid, and you will be passing those blind spots along to your students, denying them the potential benefits of specific postures or the satisfaction of exploring an experience on their own. You also are likely familiar with the basics of whatever approach you use and may not revisit the fundamental postures or transitions regularly. If you teach exactly as you practice, you may be omitting foundational concepts that are especially important for beginners to learn.

A better choice: Separate your personal practice from your teaching. Use your own practice and attend classes as a student to nourish yourself. When planning sequences for your classes, put your student first, keep in mind their preferences and level of experience, and create a practice to meet their unique needs.

Suggested Exercise:

What are your pitfalls?

Journal: Go through an existing sequence or recall a recent class you have taught. Did that sequence have any of the pitfalls mentioned in this chapter? If so, how might you adjust your sequence to avoid them if you were to teach this sequence again?

4

The Magical Worksheet

Now that you've evaluated your BIG WHY, your intentions, considered the context in which you're teaching, and know how to recognize common sequencing pitfalls, it's time to actually create a sequence.

The Magical Worksheet is a visual tool, like a mind map, to help organize a yoga practice. I originally created this worksheet as a framework to help me gather information and quickly plan practices for my private yoga clients. It's magical because it can be used in any context—whether you're working with an individual or planning a class—and for any style or approach to yoga. It simply catches all the most important factors to consider when planning a sequence and gives you space to write it down. Putting all this information on one sheet of paper allows you to quickly note the key postures of a practice and makes it easy to see how everything fits together.

The Magical Worksheet is based on a series of questions—many that we've already explored in the previous chapters—designed to help you identify potential postures.

Start by answering all of the numbered questions in the left hand column. Next, fill in the table in the upper right corner; this section is meant to get to the root of your practice, which you will build upon in the table below it, titled "Postures." In the "Postures" table, draft your sequence based on the information you've already written.

Let's walk through the worksheet questions in detail. Refer to the sample sequence at the end of the chapter using the Magical Worksheet.

1. What is the intention?

Remember that the first principle of creating effective sequences is beginning with a **simple intention**. Questions to consider include: What is the underlying purpose of the practice you are planning? Are you teaching a specific topic? How do you want your students to feel? What is your message?

Here are some examples to get you thinking: work towards headstand, experience the relationship between breath and movement, or relax before bedtime. In my Magical Worksheet example, my intention is exploring backbends.

2. What are the core postures?

Choose 1-3 core postures that align with your intention. These fundamental postures will serve as a foundation on which you can build preparation, counterposes, and transitions. Three is all you need, but you can also choose fewer. If you are planning a practice based on a pinnacle posture, you might have only one core posture, but if you are planning a practice with a broader scope, you will likely have three. Choosing more than three main postures makes it tricky to manage transitions and keep the practice elegant, particularly if you have limited time in which to do the practice. In my Magical Worksheet example, the core postures use different planes and intensities to explore backbends: *dhanurasana*, *salabhasana*, and *virabhadrasana*.

3. What's the context?

Remember that the context includes the time of day, class length, location, and a general statement about the group or person you are working with. You can describe the practice setting: "weekly one hour drop-in class at library, no yoga props available, different group of students every week" or "home practice for competitive athlete to do in the evening after strength training." Use a brief phrase to keep yourself focused as you plan the sequence. The context for the sample sequence is an hour-long class at a fitness club, with students who are mostly middle age, middle class working folks, who likely spend much of their day sitting at desks and may spend additional time sitting in a car during their commute.

4. Student demographics and level of experience

Remember that you are in the service of your students, no matter their demographic or experience level. Practitioners' age, occupation, or lifestyle, as well as their prior yoga and movement experience should influence the postures you choose. If you have a diverse group of students with varying levels of experience, or you're not sure who will show up to a particular class, note that too.

5. What do your students WANT?

When you keep your students' favorite postures, transitions, and preferred intensity in mind, your students are more likely to enjoy the practice and be engaged with your material. As you develop rapport and trust by including things your students like, you'll be able to include what they need with more positive results.

6. What are the potential risks and things to avoid?

When you identify risks associated with particular postures, you can plan appropriate variations as well as proper preparation and compensation to make the overall sequence as safe as possible. The demographics and context of a practice can also give you insight into what to avoid. If you know in advance you'll be working with beginners with little movement experience and no access to props, you should probably avoid complex postures and transitions.

When considering which postures and transitions to omit, keep in mind what your students students don't want. Of course, students can benefit from exploring the edges of their comfort zone, but if a practice is too challenging or otherwise does not meet their expectations, students can get frustrated, give up, or shut down. So, it is important to meet your students where they are. I've created the "Slow Flow" sample sequence for students who don't like an intensely strenuous practice, so I only included simple strengthening postures with adequate time focused on relaxation towards the end of the class.

7. What else might you take into consideration?

Use this section to include any other ideas that don't fit into the other sections or boxes in the worksheet. You might note if the sequence is one of a series, the unique limitations of your students, which specific props are or are not available, a description of the room environment, or anything else is going on in your students' day. Non-yoga related logistics can be important here too: for example, the child care center closes five minutes after class so you have to make sure you end on time so your students can pick up their children. In the "Slow Flow" sample sequence I've included simple options, because those students have limited yoga experience.

Yoga Stick Figures

You'll notice throughout this book that I'm using yoga stick figures, which are my preferred way of taking yoga notes. The key anatomy of a yoga stick figure are legs, feet, spine, arms, head and nose, a dot or line that shows you which direction the head is facing. You can learn more about how to draw stick figures at my website: *yogawithflissy.com/how-to-draw-yoga-stick-figures*.

Draft Your Sequence

Once you have answered the worksheet questions, you can move the key points into the boxes on the right hand side of the worksheet and draft your sequence. Use the two-column space on the right to jot down ideas for your sequence. You can write out the names of yoga postures, use your own yoga shorthand, or use my stick figures.

Start with the core postures, which will likely go somewhere in the middle. I've noted these with stars in the sample sequence for easy reference.

Next, identify relevant **warm up and preparation** postures. When planning preparation postures, remember to work from simple to complex and from general to subtle. In the sample sequence, *vajrasana* and sun salutations are used to warm up the spine for deeper backbends. Arm movement in *trikonasana* prepares the shoulder joint for the bind in *dhanurasana*.

After you have selected your essential preparation postures, select relevant **compensation and finishing** postures. Remember that counterposes should be simpler than the peak posture or core postures. In the sample sequence, I use *apanasana*, *jatthara parivrtti* (supine twist), and *janu sirsasana* (head to knee) as counterposes.

Finishing postures help prepare the body and mind to rest in *savasana* and bring balance to the whole practice. Once you have set the core postures, preparation, and compensation, fill in the gaps using transitional postures that connect one plane to the next. You can add in simple forward bends to transition between directions of movement.

Now it's time to **finalize the sequence**. Rewrite it neatly on a fresh page so you can easily reference it when you are practicing or teaching. Here you may also choose to set the breathing cues, number of repetitions, or timing for each posture or flow. Finally, check your sequence against the sequencing principles in Chapter 1, and make sure it fits the context in which you'll be teaching or practicing it.

Suggested Exercise:

Use the Magical Worksheet to make a sequence.

Magical Worksheet Sample Sequence

Class: __Slow Flow__   **Yoga Sequence Worksheet**   Date/Time: __3/18 7pm__

1. What is the intention?
Explore backbends

2. What are the core postures?
Dhanurasana, prone backbends, virabhadrasana

3. What's the context?
Fitness club, 1 hour, middle age working folks

4. Student demographics & level of experience
Mostly middle age, some yoga experience

5. Time of day
7pm

6. Location/other notes
Fitness club, hour long class

7. What do your students WANT?
Some challenge, feel relaxed at end

8. What are the potential risks and things to avoid?
Risk to low back strain, neck strain

9. What else might you take into consideration?
Time to relax at end, beginners dropping in, warm up appropriately and have simple options

Intention	Context	Time of Day
Explore backbends	Gym, working folks	7pm 1 hr
Core Pose/Seq	**Core Pose/Seq**	**Core Pose/Seq**

20

Backbend Slow Flow Practice from Magical Worksheet

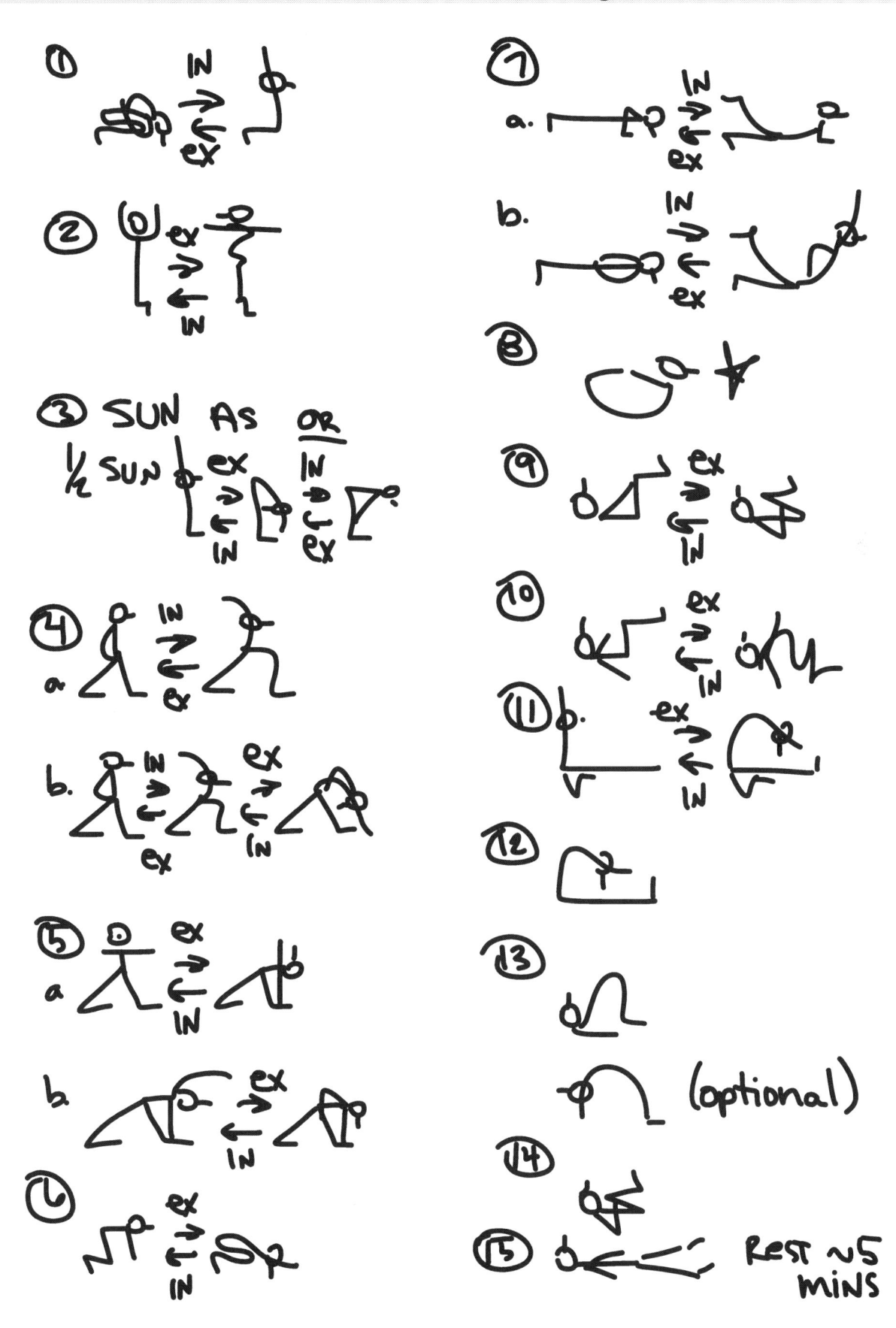

5

The Magical Outline

While the Magical Worksheet is the best tool if you need to create a sequence completely from scratch, the Magical Outline is a template for a yoga practice that follows a specific thematic arc. Use it to build sequences that follow a fairly set structure, so you can easily drop postures into a practice. Fill in postures based on your intention and adapt a practice to any style or approach.

What makes the the Magical Outline particularly useful and efficient is that the arc of the class and main transitions are already planned. This framework makes it easy to modify classes in the moment, because each section of class narrows down your posture choices to meet a specific category, for example, postures that focus on legs and hips. You can also adjust it to align with your tradition or style.

The outline breaks the practice into sections to help you to identify and create chunks of shorter sequences, which you can reuse in other practices. This structure makes it easy to see where you can plan to pepper in talking points based on your underlying intention or message. Breaking a practice into chunks also helps with time management. For a 60-minute practice, you could plan to spend five to ten minutes on each section of the practice.

I designed the The Magical Outline based on the core similarities shared between various approaches to yoga I have experienced over the years. It incorporates elements from Ashtanga Vinyasa, like sun salutations and a finishing sequence, as well as "hatha" practices rooted in alignment-based approaches such as those devised by B. K. S. Iyengar, which place an emphasis on static standing postures and seated stretches. The sample sequence at the end of this section is a basic flow class inspired by Ashtanga Vinyasa.

The Magical Outline breaks a sequence into the following sections:

Centering

The first few minutes of a yoga practice are devoted to centering. Centering includes bringing awareness to the present moment and preparing the mind to focus on the yoga practice. In this section, you might include an introduction to the theme of the class, guide students to a comfortable position, practice breath awareness, teach *ujjayi pranayama*, chant, or lead a short meditation. Most yoga practices begin in a seated position, but you might choose to start standing or lying down, depending on your overall plan for the practice.

Opening Sequence

The primary intention for an opening sequence is joint mobilization, a crucial element of warming up the body in preparation for more complex or strenuous movements. It should include simple, dynamic movements rather than static stretches to most effectively warm up the joints and muscles. The sample sequence has three different movements on the hands and knees to warm up the spine, hips, and shoulders. Depending on how much time you have, this section could be a series of three to five simple movements. Many yoga classes begin with some variation of cat/cow or *cakravakasana*, which is certainly appropriate because both are simple ways to mobilize the spine. Depending on the style or tradition of yoga, you might also use the opening sequence to introduce the relationship between breath and movement. Regardless of your approach or tradition, the opening sequence should begin to develop the mind-body connection that is fundamental to the practice of yoga.

Spine

As the title implies, this section focuses on the musculature around the spine. You can also use it as a continuation of the opening sequence. In an Ashtanga Vinyasa or flow style practice, you'd use sun salutation A and its variations. Traditional sun salutations focus on flexion and extension of the spine through the repetition of standing forward bends and *urdhva mukha svanasana* (upward facing dog). I tend to incorporate simple prone backbends here because they are less strenuous than *urdhva mukha svanasana* and they provide the back strengthening benefits many people need due to sedentary habits. So, this section may use sun salutation A or a variation, or may be a sequence of several postures that focus on general movement of the spine. Refer back to your main intention with the practice for ideas on what you might introduce in this section. For example, if your practice focuses on twists, you may begin to incorporate a simple supine or standing twist to get started.

Hips & Legs

Once you've warmed up the main joints and musculature around the spine, you'll move onto the hips and legs. In an Ashtanga Vinyasa or flow class, this includes sun salutation B as well as standing postures. In a hatha class, you might only do standing postures. You may spend the bulk of a practice focusing on this section because standing postures are so beneficial for strengthening and stretching the large muscles of the legs, hips, and back, as well as developing balance and overall coordination. A restorative, yin, or gentle class might include dynamic or static postures that focus on the legs and hips but may not necessarily build the same heat.

Featured Topic

After the body is well warmed up and the mind is focused on the practice—about halfway or two-thirds of the way through—you can introduce the featured topic. In a group class context, it is the best time to introduce a new concept or posture. I sometimes call this section "Teach a thing!" At least one of your core postures should go here. In the sample sequence I am using this section to teach *drishti* (eye gaze) to help with balance, and so my core postures, *hasta padangusthasana* (hand to big toe) and *ardha baddha padmasana* (half bound lotus)—both single leg balances—go here. If you imagine that the practice is shaped like a bell curve, the featured topic will be the peak.

Seated and Supine

At this point, you have done a bulk of the strenuous work and the muscles are warm, which makes it the best time in the sequence to focus on flexibility through static seated and supine stretches. This section may begin to incorporate counterposes or compensation for core postures, or it may focus on flexibility of the spine and hips in a more general way. The seated sequence in the primary series of Ashtanga Vinyasa is a good example of this section, and I have borrowed a few postures for the sample sequence. In sequencing a yin or restorative practice, it is appropriate to put the more complex or more intense stretches in this section.

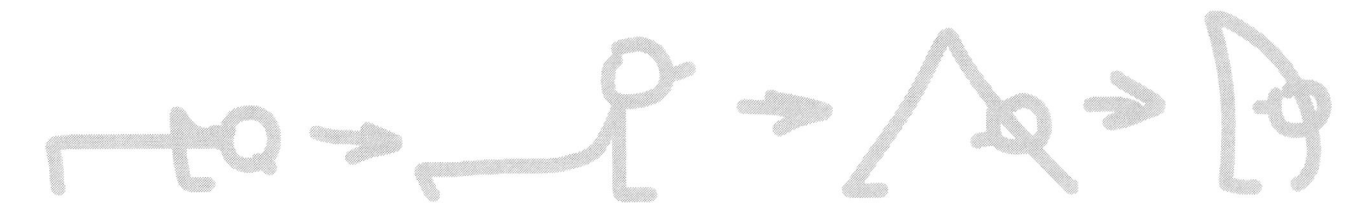

Finishing Sequence

The finishing sequence will compensate for any residual stress or potential risks from postures used earlier in the practice and prepare the body for relaxation. *Dwi pada pittham* and *viminasana* (a prone backbend with hip abduction and adduction) are both ideal postures for stabilization after a practice that demands intense flexibility, whereas seated forward bends may be more appropriate to compensate for an extremely energizing practice. Simple supine postures such as *jatthara parivrtti* and *apanasana* are useful to wind down the practice just before resting in *savasana*, because they are gentle ways to release tension and many students enjoy them. You could also incorporate the traditional Ashtanga Vinyasa "finishing sequence," which includes *sirsasana* and *sarvangasana*, or use a variation.

Relaxation and Meditation

A yoga practice differs from other movement practices in that it begins and ends with quiet contemplation. Traditionally, a yoga practice ends with a few minutes in *savasana* to rest and integrate the effects of the practice. You might want to note how long you plan to spend in *savasana*, if you plan to use some kind of guided meditation or include *pranayama*, or any other talking points you might use to wrap up your class.

Adapting for Other Styles

As with all the content presented, this outline is a tool for you to use and adapt to suit your needs. Some schools of yoga have a similar progression that may have prone backbends, followed by core work, then arm balances after the standing hip/leg sequence. Some traditions of yoga are completely separate from the Krishnamacharya lineage where both Ashtanga Vinyasa and Iyengar-inspired alignment methods originate, in which case, the progression may be quite different than the one in the Magical Outline. For example, yin and restorative practices are not often taught with the Magical Outline arc; however, applying the concepts therein can provide a structure where proper preparation and compensation are included and so that the practice is balanced overall.

Look for patterns in the sequences of any school of yoga and identify logical sections where the postures can be interchangeable. You can use this template to consider the arc of a class and identify the arc of a practice in your tradition.

Suggested Exercise:

Use the Magical Outline to create a yoga sequence.

Magical Outline Sample Sequence

Class: __AM Flow__   Yoga Sequence Outline   Date/Time: __9/12__

Intention	Context	Time of Day	Core Pose	Core Pose	Core Pose
inspired by AV, ujjayi and drishti	at gym, 20s-30s, experienced	8:30 AM	SUN SALUTES	*(sketch)*	*(sketch)*

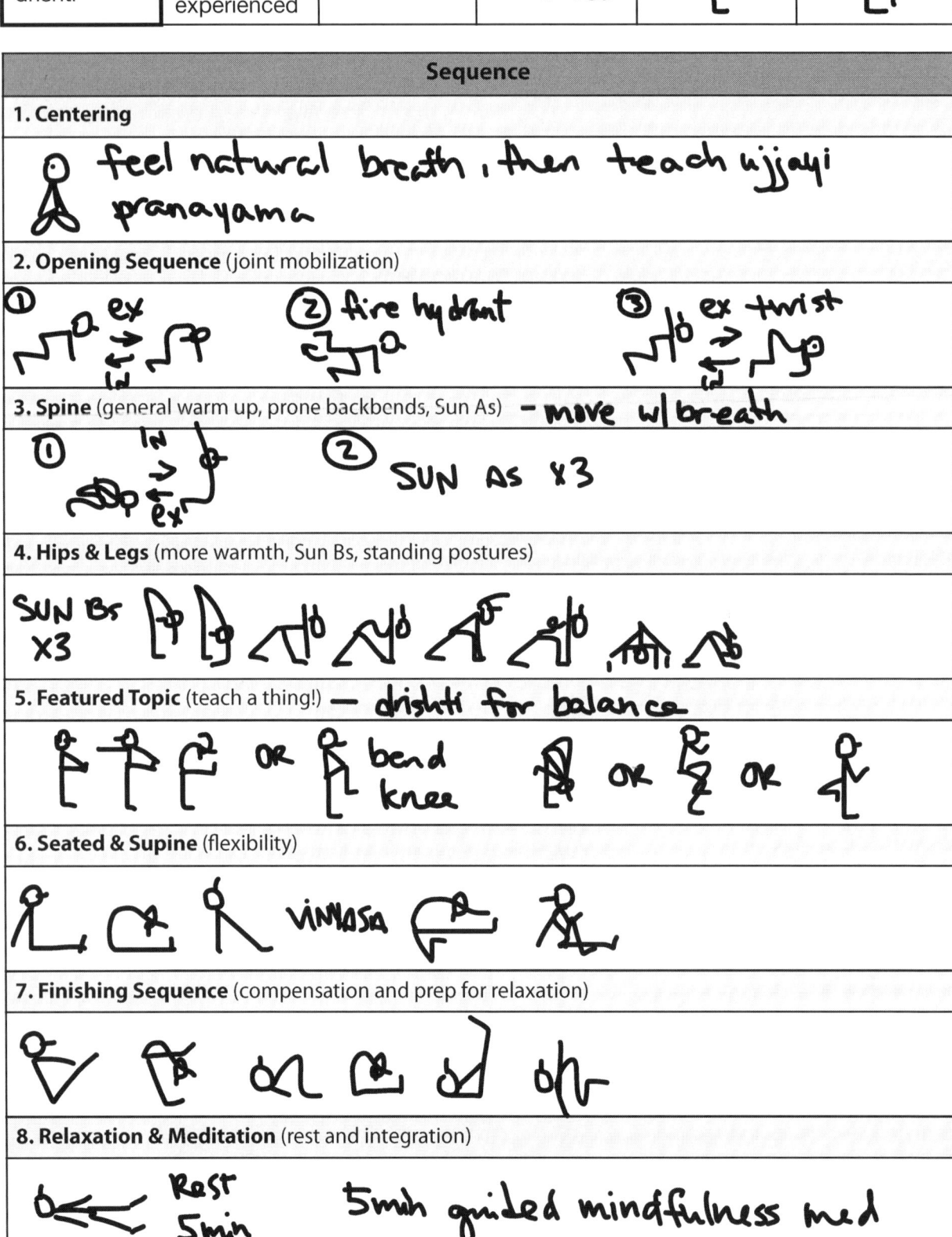

Sequence

1. Centering
feel natural breath, then teach ujjayi pranayama

2. Opening Sequence (joint mobilization)
① ex   ② fire hydrant   ③ ex twist

3. Spine (general warm up, prone backbends, Sun As) — move w/ breath
① IN / ex   ② SUN As x3

4. Hips & Legs (more warmth, Sun Bs, standing postures)
SUN Bs x3

5. Featured Topic (teach a thing!) — drishti for balance
or bend knee   or   or

6. Seated & Supine (flexibility)
vinyasa

7. Finishing Sequence (compensation and prep for relaxation)

8. Relaxation & Meditation (rest and integration)
Rest 5min   5min guided mindfulness med

6

Yoga Court

After you've created sequences using the Magical Worksheet and/or the Magical Outline, it's time to defend your sequence in Yoga Court.

Yoga Court is a concept introduced to me by my teacher, Gary Kraftsow, as a way to evaluate, check, and adjust a sequence according to a set of principles and questions. You don't need to actually contact anyone else to go to Yoga Court, because the only "judges" are the questions that invite you to examine your choices. You should be able to defend your sequence by analyzing it based on the principles we've established as well as answering some yes or no questions. Fortunately, the "judges" are lenient and are primarily looking for the why behind what you are teaching!

First, check that your sequence adheres to the yoga sequencing principles:

1. Start with a (simple!) intention
2. Apply general fitness rules
3. Be aware of planes
4. Use proper preparation and compensation
5. Move from simple to complex
6. Consider risks vs. benefits

Does your sequence adhere to the principles? If not, why not? What can you do to bring your sequence into better alignment with the above principles?

Then, answer the following questions to dig deeper into your sequence:

1. **Do the sequence and included postures reflect the overall intention?**

Make sure the postures you have included, particularly the core postures, are relevant to the overall intention.

2. **Is there appropriate transition between planes?**

Appropriate transitions are based on the principle that you should pass through kneeling when moving up or down from the floor, and with consideration for the context in which you'll be teaching. Though it may be technically correct to go from a single leg balance to a kneeling lunge to *urdhva dhanurasana* and back again, that transition might be impossible for those with limited mobility. With that in mind, remember to pass through kneeling when moving from standing to supine or vice versa. When checking your sequence for appropriate transition between planes, it's also useful to evaluate how much transitioning up and down is happening and consider if it is more efficient to rearrange things for fewer transitions.

3. **Is there use of forward bends to transition between directions of movement?**

Use simple forward bends like *uttanasana*, *balasana*, *paschimatanasana* (seated forward bend), and *apanasana* to stretch the back when changing direction from lateral bends, twists, and backbends. Make sure there is adequate compensation before moving to the next posture or sequence in your practice.

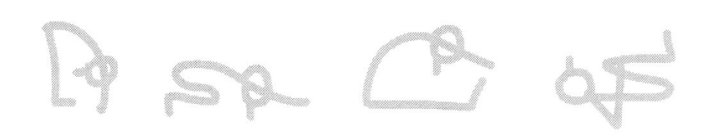

4. **Does this sequence fit the context in which you'll teach it?**

A sequence may be technically correct but not appropriate for the context where you are teaching. Do you have all the props or equipment you need? Do the postures selected align with the experience level and ability of your students? Have you considered adaptations and variations of postures to use if you need to make changes once you're in class?

5. **Is the sequence efficient and elegant?**

This last question addresses the art of sequencing and is subjective. An efficient and elegant practice will have minimal transitions and include only the most relevant postures.

Every practitioner will have their own sense of flow, so make sure you actually do your planned sequence to see how it feels. Remember that if you're planning to teach the sequence, that you'll have to consider your students unique abilities and limitations. With practice and experience, you will understand what postures make sense together for your own practice and style, as well as what sequences are a good fit for your students.

Suggested Exercise:

Using the Yoga Court Checklist in the Appendix, evaluate one of your own yoga sequences.

7

Applications

Once you've worked with both the Magical Worksheet and the Magical Outline to determine what works best for how you plan, practice, and teach, you'll probably want to dig a little deeper into how to apply the sequencing guidelines. So I've included a few more suggestions about how to use the tools in this book for self-reflection, developing yourself as a teacher, and for creating a library of practices to make class planning more efficient.

Long Term Planning

Whether you are planning a session that spans several weeks or are teaching ongoing classes, set a simple intention that spans the long term. I recommend using the Magical Worksheet to better understand the context and demographics of the people you will be teaching, then, instead of setting three core postures, note a few main concepts and a handful of postures that support your ideas. For each class in the series, set a new simple intention that teaches one element of the long term goal. You can use the Magical Worksheet or the Magical Outline to create sequences for each class in the series. Refer to Chapter 9: Pinnacle Posture: Creating a Series for an example of how to use the Magical Outline to create sequences for a series.

Easily Adjust Existing Material

Even though many yoga teachers feel pressure to create creative new flows every class, students learn best when key material is repeated. They'll feel at ease knowing in general what to expect week-to-week. Embrace repetition by keeping a few chunks of class the same, such as repeating an opening or finishing sequence several weeks in a row. Use variations on core postures and teach different elements of the same posture week-to-week to introduce variety while reinforcing core concepts. When you are teaching a series, work from simple to complex over a longer period of time by building on concepts as classes progresses and/or working on more challenging variations on postures.

Keep Up With Ongoing Teaching Demands

Many yoga teachers teach multiple classes per week and struggle to keep up with the planning demands. An efficient way to plan is to work with a single intention and then adapt that sequence based on the context and time of day. (See the Appendix for an example of a power flow versus a gentle sequence, both based on the same intention.) You can also teach the same sequence multiple times and shift the focus of your instruction to highlight a different concept or technique. Again, the repetition of the sequence will help practitioners solidify their understanding of the postures, transitions, and concepts.

Build Your Collection

One of the benefits of taking the time to plan and write down sequences is that you'll begin to build a collection. Keep a journal of the sequences you create. Make sure to note the date of the practice and test out the sequences yourself. When you teach, note any changes you made to the planned sequence, and take a few moments to write what went well and what to do differently next time. When you have a collection of sequences, you can easily reuse them as is, swap out sections, or adapt them for different contexts. Look for patterns in your sequences to identify short flows that work well. Through this work, not only will you develop your voice as a teacher, but you'll also create a diverse range of material that you can apply in various lesson plans and contexts.

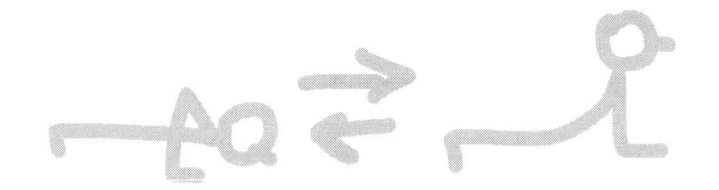

Working in Specific Contexts

Effective yoga teachers can teach diverse groups of students and meet their unique needs, but if you are already a yoga teacher, you understand that doing so can be quite challenging. Whether you are working one-on-one or with a group, you will need to think about not only how your students are different from one another, but also how certain sequencing approaches will serve them best. If you're working with a student in a private session, you'll be able to narrow your focus. Group classes can be tricky, because of various experience levels or inconsistent attendance. Thankfully, group classes are usually separated by style such as restorative or flow, or by levels of experience, and so we can apply the sequencing principles and tools to plan a class to fit what students may expect based on a class description.

Planning for Mixed Levels

The reality of most group classes is that they are all mixed levels! People often take yoga classes at the time that is convenient for them, regardless of whether or not the classes are appropriate for their experience level. In addition, everyone is susceptible to injury and illness—even the most experienced yoga practitioners—so it is important to consider accessibility in every class you plan and teach so that everyone has the ability to participate equally.

When planning a mixed level class, proper use of preparation postures is key to teach practitioners fundamental movement techniques and lay the foundation for understanding individual postures. Build up to holding static postures by beginning with dynamic movement, and experiment with how and when you'll stay longer in postures to control the intensity. Revisit the principles of working from simple to complex and from general to subtle to deliver layers of information and provide options for students to work at their own pace. Remember you can vary the load and change planes to adjust the intensity of postures, and even have students working in different planes as needed.

Your planned sequence is just that—a plan—and it is subject to change based on who you are teaching and what is happening in the moment. As you are teaching, deliver information in a thoughtful progression, beginning with the breath cue (if appropriate to the style you are teaching), a clear direction about the movement, and finally any details (a metaphor, a refinement about alignment, etc.). Then, observe how your students are embodying your instruction and respond appropriately. Be open to changing your plan, repeating things, or skipping some postures altogether to meet the needs of your students that day.

Sequencing for Beginner Students

Beginners are new to the principles and movements of yoga postures and philosophies, even if they have other fitness or movement experience. Many yoga teachers learn to teach yoga classes to their peers, which is not at all a realistic representation of teaching in the real world! Teachers sometimes lose track of what makes a class appropriate for beginners and how to meet the needs of folks who are just getting started with yoga or movement practices. It's highly likely that you'll be teaching students who are new to yoga, because people continually seek out yoga classes for both physical wellness and stress relief.

Here are some sequencing tips for teaching beginners:

- Remember to **keep it simple** and begin with the most fundamental versions of postures.

- **Minimize transitions** up and down from the floor.

- **Use lots of repetition** to teach core concepts and reinforce understanding of basic movements and techniques.

- **Allow adequate time to rest** and transition between postures.

- **Allow for omissions.** Beginners often need more instruction, repetition, and transitions, so plan which postures can be cut out should you run short on time.

- **Plan adaptations** to simplify postures, vary the load, or use props to accommodate beginners who may have limited mobility or strength.

One-on-One

The advantage and fun of working one-on-one with yoga practitioners is that you get to co-create a practice with them based on their unique goals, needs, and feedback about what postures and approaches to practice they prefer. The sequencing principles and the Magical Worksheet are essential tools for private yoga instruction. When you understand the purposes, benefits, and applications of specific postures and practice as well as the art and science of sound sequencing, you are in a position of expertise to help people do the exact practice to suit their individual needs.

Restorative/Yin

Though restorative and yin yoga are different practices with unique purposes, what they have in common is that they break the rules of general fitness principles by being quiet practices that consist primarily of static positions held for longer periods of time. That being said, if you teach yin or restorative yoga, consider using some gentle, dynamic movement to address the common tension, agitation, and stiffness the general public carries with them into a yoga class. Because these practices are nuanced with powerful effects on the nervous system, pay special attention to the arc of the class so that the overall practice will create the energetic effect you intend.

Vinyasa/Flow

When planning a vinyasa or flow class, each flow sequence should adhere to the principles we've established. Think of each flow as a mini-practice that progresses from simple to complex and incorporates proper preparation and compensation. At first, you might feel like this approach creates extra work for you, but soon you'll be able to swap flows in and out of larger practices to create infinite variations, and it will improve the overall safety of your practices by minimizing unnecessary risk or stress to the joints. Of course, the practice as a whole should also adhere to the sequencing principles.

Other Traditions

Even though my background is rooted in the teachings and lineage of Krishnamacharya, there are, of course, many other traditions of yoga, some of which have completely different approaches from what I offer. Use whatever principles and tools are relevant to your own approach, adapt them as you like, and feel free to set aside whatever is not useful.

Final Thoughts

As you use these tools I invite you to be curious about your own practice, creative about crafting sequences, and analytical about sequences by asking yourself, your peers, and your teachers why they choose to put things where they do. Sometimes the answer may be "because it's always done this way," which is a valid answer; tradition is an important facet of yoga. Just as if you were to take a trip from one city to another there are many different modes of transportation and routes you could take depending on your priorities, there are many ways to create a satisfying, safe, effective yoga practice, so enjoy the process of exploring your yoga practice through sequencing.

9

Sample Sequences

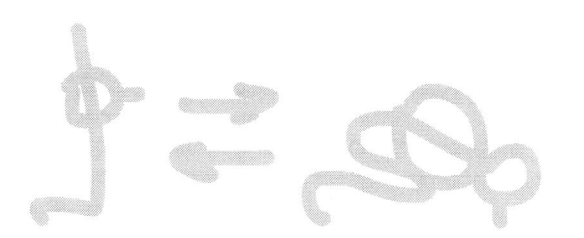

Now that you understand the principles of yoga sequencing, let's look at some examples. You can think of these sample sequences as "Yoga Sequence Recipes." They demonstrate how to craft a sequence based on a simple intention and a generalized context. Feel free to practice and teach these sequences as is, or change them to match your personal style or different contexts. In addition to the sequences themselves, I've written a brief description of why I created each one. I've also indicated the core postures with stars.

Suggested Exercise:

Take one of these sample sequences and rework it for a specific context.

1: A Sequence to Address Poor Posture

Many people come to yoga to improve their posture or address back pain (often a result of chronic poor posture). Most people need to relieve the physical effects of stress, such as muscular tension around the back or neck, as well as the mental/ psychological effects, like racing thoughts and poor sleep patterns, by settling the nervous system. A sequence addressing these common issues would include back strengthening, stretching the front of the hips, and mobilizing the neck and shoulders.

In this sample sequence, I've included *virabhadrasana* (#3), *salabhasana* (#7), and *eka pada ustrasana* (low lunge, #8) as the core postures. The version of *virabhadrasana* (#3) included in this practice incorporates protraction and retraction of the scapulae to address thoracic and shoulder mobility; it also stretches and strengthens the muscles around the legs, hips, and back. I have placed *virabhadrasana* before *salabhasana* (#7) because it is a little less strenuous than *salabhasana* due to the upright position of the torso and therefore less work against gravity. *Salabhasana* also incorporates shoulder mobility, though any prone backbend is an excellent choice to strengthen the musculature around the low back. After preparation through those two backends, *eka pada ustrasana* (#8) provides deeper stretch for the hip flexors and whole front side of the body.

I've filled out the practice with some arm sweeps and head turns in twists (#5, #10) to further address neck and shoulder tension, and balanced out the movements with forward bends (#2, 4, 6, 9, 11, 12) for compensation and to stretch the low back.

This sequence is a simple, balanced Viniyoga sequence that would be appropriate for most levels of experience, so long as practitioners are able to get up and down from the floor and be on their knees.

Address Poor Posture

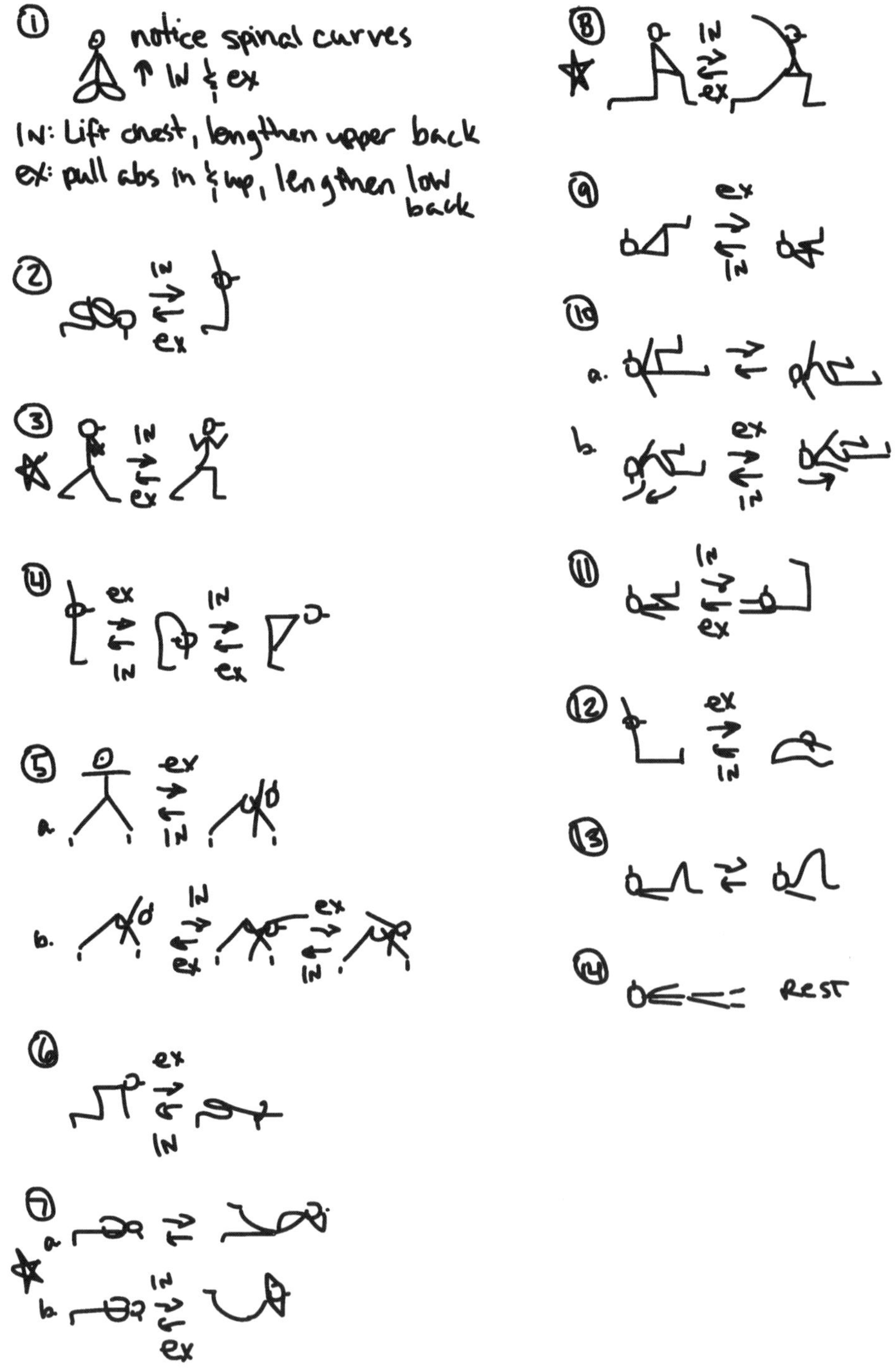

① notice spinal curves ↑ IN & ex

IN: Lift chest, lengthen upper back
ex: pull abs in & up, lengthen low back

②

③

④

⑤ a.
b.

⑥

⑦ a.
b.

⑧

⑨

⑩ a.
b.

⑪

⑫

⑬

⑭ Rest

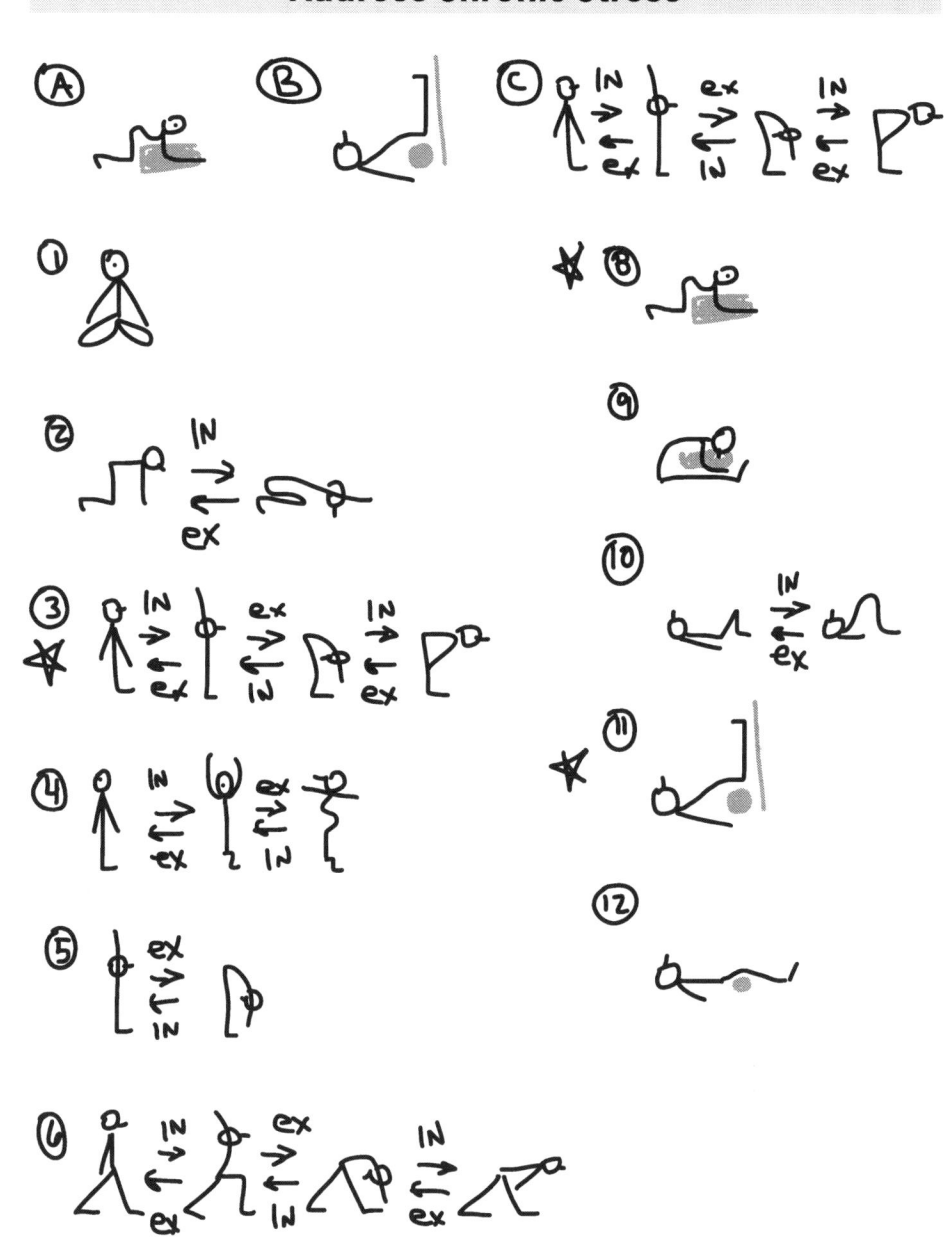

2: A Sequence to Address Chronic Stress

Many people come to yoga hoping to find some respite from their busy lives. And, of course, there are many ways to address chronic stress through yoga. Most people need to relieve the physical effects of stress, such as muscular tension around the back or neck, as well as the mental/psychological effects, like racing thoughts and poor sleep patterns, by settling the nervous system. Due to the busyness of modern culture, many people have difficulty slowing down or sitting still, so this sequence begins more active and then shifts to more still and restorative.

The core postures for this sequence incorporate both dynamic and restorative postures: a half sun salutation (#3), a prone twist on a bolster (#8), and *viparita karani* (legs up the wall, #11).

Placing the half sun salutations towards the beginning of the practice warms up the spine and hips to prepare for the postures held on the floor, and the sequence of moving with the breath establishes a solid mind-body connection for the whole practice. The twisting variation of *tadasana* (#4) gives the mind a job to do by focusing on balance. *Parsvatanasana* (#6) further prepares the hips, back, and hamstrings to hold a seated supported forward bend. The prone twist (#8) is both a forward bend and twist, and the support of the bolster makes it particularly restful. A supported *paschimatanasana* (#9) and *viparita karani* (#11)—our final core posture—calm the nervous system, and are excellent postures to put towards the end of the practice.

This sequence is particularly useful for people rushing from work to yoga in the evening as it includes both active and passive practice, and can easily be modified to suit individuals with varying degrees of experience and mobility through the use of props.

Address Chronic Stress

3: A Sequence to Address Dysfunctional Breathing Patterns

One of the challenges of teaching breath centric yoga practices is helping practitioners understand the relationship between breath and movement, and teaching more refined control of the breath that can benefit their breath throughout the day. Many people go about their day taking shallow breaths due to poor posture, which could contribute to feelings of lethargy, or they have patterns of holding their breath, which might contribute to stress or anxiety. The amazing thing about the breath is that it is both an automatic fact of life and a conscious action that can be controlled to improve technique for moving in and out of yoga postures as well as benefit the nervous system.

The core postures for this sequence are *uttanasana* (#9), *trikonasana* (#10) with arm sweeps, and *jathara parivrtti* (#4). The practice begins with coordinating breath with movement of the arms and feet. Then, it focuses on using the exhale to create the twist in *jathara parivrtti* (#4). Next, there is a series of postures to compensate for the twist and transition to standing. *Uttanasana* (#9) is ideal for working on the relationship between breath and movement because it is a big, full body movement and even experienced yoga practitioners can improve the relationship between the hips and spinal curves by refining the transition from standing to the forward bend and back. The arm sweeps in *trikonasana* (#10) help focus attention on the inhale and facilitate expansion of the ribcage so practitioners can take even deeper breaths.

This sequence begins supine and transitions to standing to seated, which makes it a useful practice for the the morning because it gradually builds to a more active practice. Because this is a breath centric practice, it could be used as a preparation for *pranayama* by incorporating breath adaptions for lengthening various parts of the breath.

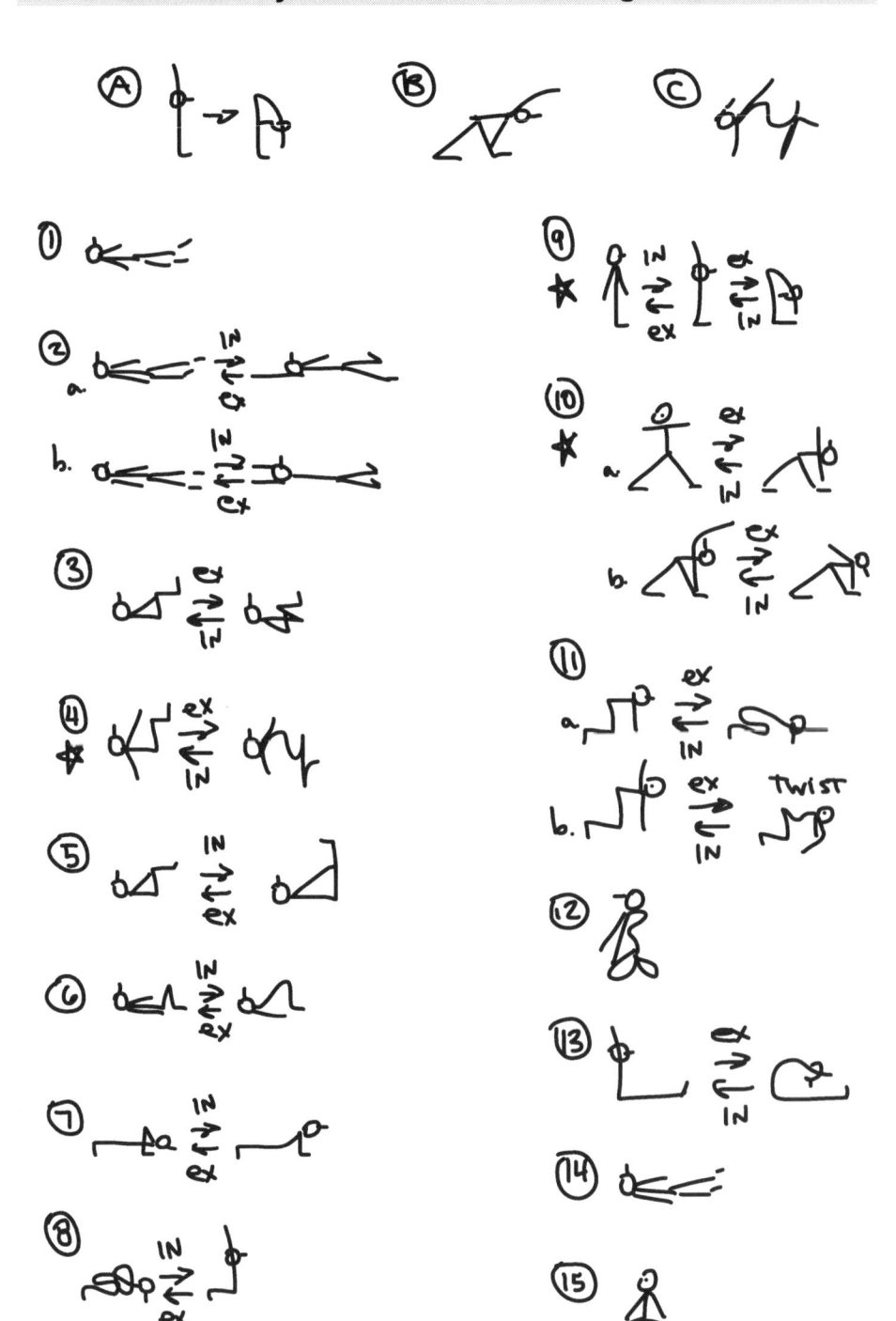

Address Dysfunctional Breathing Patterns

4: A Sequence to Build up to a Pinnacle Posture

A pinnacle posture is one that is challenging or difficult, often requiring additional practice, flexibility, balance, or strength to achieve. When planning a practice for a pinnacle posture, select one or two other core postures that support your main one. In the fitness world, this is called the principle of specificity: you train for your goals by doing related activities. For example, if you were training to run a marathon, you'd include running, sprinting, and endurance in your exercise sessions, but not, for example, swimming. We use the same concept here.

The pinnacle posture in this sequence is *parsva bakasana* (side crow, #14); the twisting variation of *adho mukha svanasana* (#9) and *ardha matsyendrasana* (seated twist, #13) are preparatory postures. When we break down *parsva bakasana* into its essential elements, we see that it is an arm balance with a twist, so this sequence includes core and upper body strengthening through sun salutations (#4) and the twisting variation of *adho mukha svanasana* (#9) as well as lots of twists (#7, #11, #13). I've also included the twisting version of *navasana* (boat, #15) as a challenge and for further core conditioning. The practice ends with compensation for twisting through a *pascimatanasana* (#16) and stabilization for the hips and low back (#17, 18).

This sequence is a strenuous, flowing practice for more experienced practitioners.

Pinnacle Posture: Creating a Series

Most people will need more than just one practice to execute a pinnacle posture safely or successfully, which presents an excellent opportunity for planning a series of sequences to help them get there. When planning a series, first choose your overall intention, then identify how you will support that intention in each class. The Magical Outline is particularly useful for organizing series of classes so that you can easily see the arc of a class and choose what is best to repeat.

In the following example, I used the Magical Outline to craft a series of sequences to prepare for *sirsasana*.

Week one focuses on general mobility and stability. The core postures are *navasana* to build core strength, *virabhadrasana* to mobilize upper back and shoulders, and *supta padangusthasana* to prepare for *sarvangasana* and *sirsasana* through a simpler inversion. You'll see that I've circled the postures that are repeated every week. Repeating fundamental postures reinforces important concepts and techniques and allows students to evaluate their progress over time.

Week two revisits the core postures introduced in week one and introduces dolphin as a core posture to further develop stability and upper body strength for *sirsasana*.

Week three repeats the opening sequence from week two and introduces a variation to *virabhadrasana* for scapular mobility. I've added a challenge to dolphin pose by transitioning in and out of forearm plank. In this sequence, I also introduce *sarvangasana* as the second core posture, because it is both the traditional counterpose to *sirsasana* and its broader base makes it an easier balance than headstand.

Finally, week four is a culmination of all the prior weeks as it repeats the opening sequence from week one and the full spinal sequence from week three. The hip and leg sequence incorporates all the standing postures used as preparation for the neck and shoulders and core stability. Finally, dolphin pose or *sirsasana* are offered as the pinnacle posture, before winding down the practice with a finishing sequence that includes *sarvangasana*.

I planned this series as an evening practice for a general intermediate group of practitioners. Though *sirsasana* and *sarvangasana* are pinnacle postures, the remainder of the practice is not overly complex or strenuous and therefore appropriate for a fairly diverse group, providing that options are given for those who are not able or prefer not to practice the riskier variations of the inversions included.

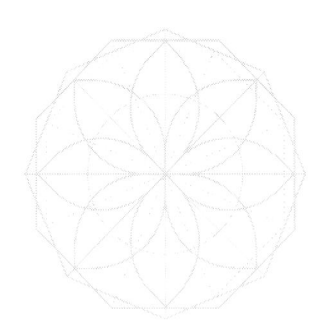

Pinnacle Posture Long Term Prep

Class: **HEADSTAND 1**   Yoga Sequence Outline   Date/Time: **wk 1**

Intention	Context	Time of Day	Core Pose	Core Pose	Core Pose
mobility & stability	4-wk series	7 pm	*(sketch)*	*(sketch)*	*(sketch)*

Sequence

1. Centering

IN: lift chest
ex: abs in   Breath will move body through practice

2. Opening Sequence (joint mobilization)

3. Spine (general warm up, prone backbends, Sun As)

SUN As x 3

4. Hips & Legs (more warmth, Sun Bs, standing postures)

5. Featured Topic (teach a thing!)

6. Seated & Supine (flexibility)

7. Finishing Sequence (compensation and prep for relaxation)

8. Relaxation & Meditation (rest and integration)

Class: **HEADSTAND 2**   Yoga Sequence Outline   Date/Time: **wk 2**

Intention	Context	Time of Day	Core Pose	Core Pose	Core Pose
core strength	4-wk series	7pm	(pose sketch)	(pose sketch)	

Sequence

1. Centering

↑IN ↓ex   ON ex' ABS IN & UP to engage CORE

2. Opening Sequence (joint mobilization)

(sketches with IN/ex notations)

3. Spine (general warm up, prone backbends, Sun As)

IN → ex →
ex ← IN ←   SUN As x3

4. Hips & Legs (more warmth, Sun Bs, standing postures)

SUN Bs x3   (triangle sketch)

5. Featured Topic (teach a thing!)

(sketches) (W1) ex→ IN↑ IN→ ex↓ ex→ ←IN

6. Seated & Supine (flexibility)

(sketches)

7. Finishing Sequence (compensation and prep for relaxation)

(W1)   (sketches)   IN→ ←ex

8. Relaxation & Meditation (rest and integration)

(savasana sketch)

Class: **Headstand 3** Yoga Sequence Outline Date/Time: **Wk 3**

Intention	Context	Time of Day	Core Pose	Core Pose	Core Pose
(headstand sketch)	4-wk series	7pm	*(headstand sketch)*	*(triangle sketch)*	

Sequence

1. Centering

↑IN ↓ex
check in w/how body feels

2. Opening Sequence (joint mobilization)

3. Spine (general warm up, prone backbends, Sun As)

Sun As × 3

4. Hips & Legs (more warmth, Sun Bs, standing postures)

5. Featured Topic (teach a thing!)

6. Seated & Supine (flexibility)

7. Finishing Sequence (compensation and prep for relaxation)

8. Relaxation & Meditation (rest and integration)

Class: **HEADSTAND 4** Yoga Sequence Outline Date/Time: **wk 4**

Intention	Context	Time of Day	Core Pose	Core Pose	Core Pose
🙆	4-wk series	7pm	🙆	🙆	🙆

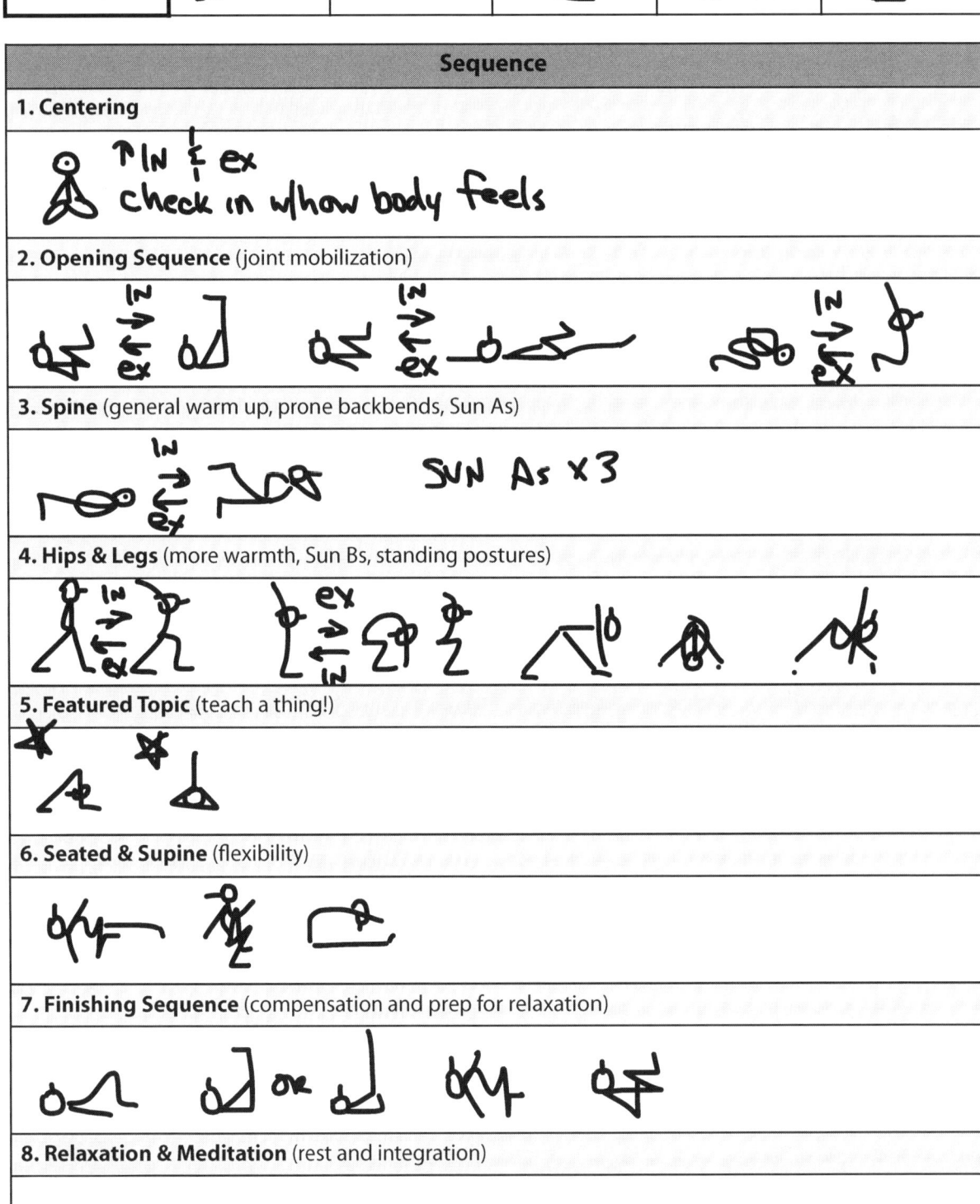

Sequence

1. Centering

↑IN ↓ex
check in w/how body feels

2. Opening Sequence (joint mobilization)

(W1)

3. Spine (general warm up, prone backbends, Sun As)

(W3) SUN As x 3

4. Hips & Legs (more warmth, Sun Bs, standing postures)

5. Featured Topic (teach a thing!)

6. Seated & Supine (flexibility)

(W3)

7. Finishing Sequence (compensation and prep for relaxation)

or

8. Relaxation & Meditation (rest and integration)

42

5: A Sequence to Explore a Posture in Different Ways

A simple way to get creative with your asana practice is to experiment with a familiar posture in various orientations. This sample sequence is an intermediate level vinyasa practice that explores *vrksasana* (tree). The core postures feature the traditional, single leg standing balance version of *vrksasana* (#10), as well as a supine version (#2), and a variation of side plank (#11).

The opening sequence includes some mobility for the low back and hips before holding the supine version of *vrksasana* (#2). Then, there is more intense warm up through sun salutations and a standing sequence focusing on balance and hip abduction to prepare for the traditional version of *vrksasana* (#10), followed by a variation in side plank (#11b).

Note that the progression of the variations of *vrksasana* go from least strenuous to most strenuous. I have also included *janu sirsasana* (#14), which has the same leg position as *vrksasana*, as well as some standing postures, as a way to explore just one element of the core posture through related positions.

Explore a Posture in Various Orientations

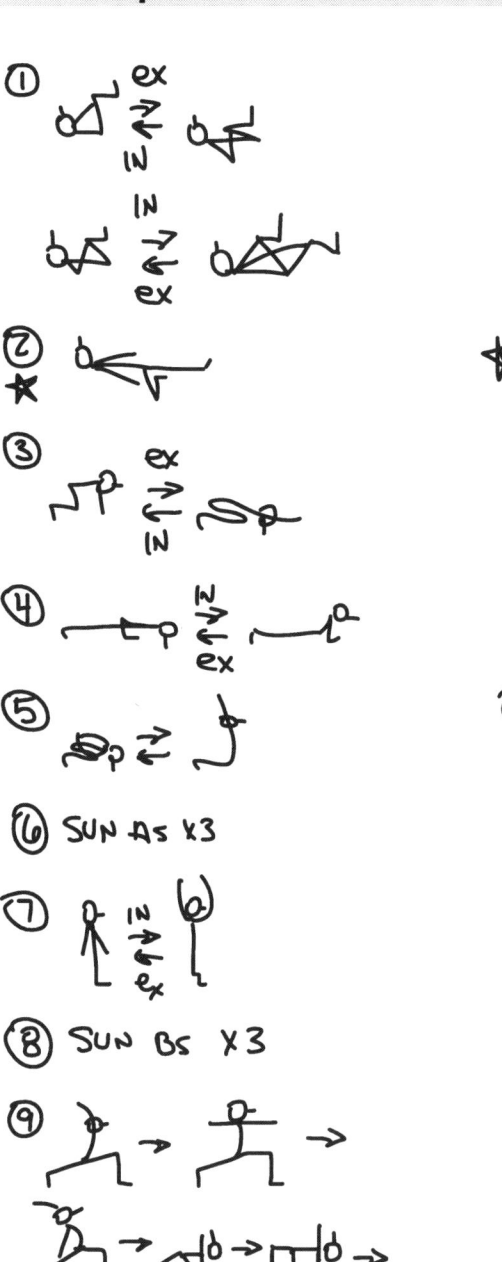

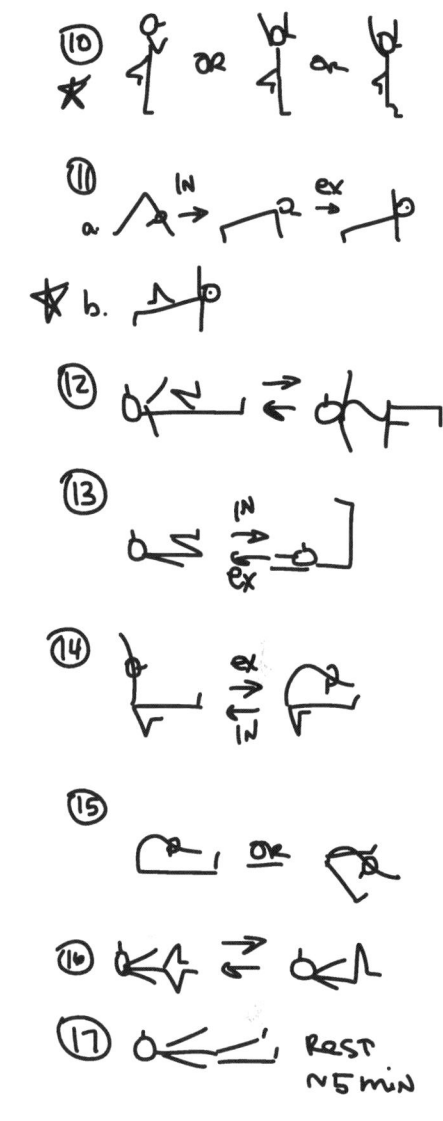

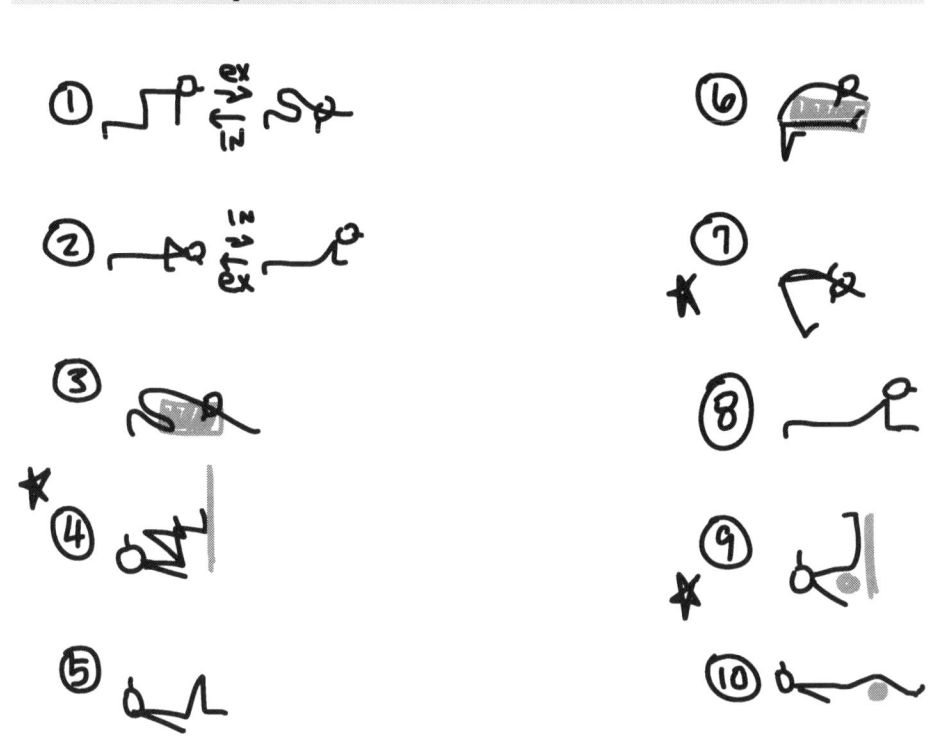

6: A Sequence to Explore a Direction of Movement

Direction of movement refers to anatomical direction, such as flexion or extension, which is the same no matter where you are oriented in space. You may choose to explore movement along an anatomical plane (such as the sagittal plane) or a direction of movement of the spine (such as twisting or lateral bending) to teach a general understanding of anatomy. Teaching a single direction of movement can also help students sense the specific effects of that movement by practicing one technique in detail. When exploring a direction of movement, it is important to remember that the practice should still be balanced and any potential strain from repetitive movement or long held positions should be compensated through use of counterposes and simple forward bends.

For this sequence, I've selected supine figure four (#4), *upavista konasana* (wide leg forward bend, #7), and *viparita karani* (#9) as core postures to explore different orientations, leg positions, and intensities of forward bending. Though the focus is on longer held positions, the practice begins with simple dynamic movement (#1, 2) and incorporates backbends (#2, #8) and rest (#5) to balance out the practice. Support under the knees is suggested in *savasana* (#10) to alleviate any residual tension in the low back.

This primarily static sample sequence could be used for a yin or restorative class that explores forward bends. You'll notice that though the practice focuses on forward bending direction, it also includes backbends and periods of rest for compensation.

Explore a Direction of Movement

7: A Sequence to Explore a Joint

One of the functions of asana practice is to explore alignment of the body to prepare for seated meditation as well as to support overall day-to-day wellness. You might teach a practice focused on a particular joint to help students understand that joint's function and promote stability and appropriate range of motion. When using a sequence to explore a joint you could explore the ways it can move, stability, mobility, or how it behaves when bearing weight versus unloaded.

This sample sequence explores shoulder mobility. Core postures explore various functions of the shoulder joint through variations of *virabhadrasana* (#6), *trikonasana* (#8), and *garudasana* (eagle, #10). Due to the intensity of focus on shoulder movements in this practice, it is most appropriate for practitioners without any known shoulder or neck injuries, otherwise it is a balanced practice of moderate intensity.

The sequence begins by introducing shoulder flexion and extension versus abduction and adduction in postures #1 through #5. Then, in *virabhadrasana* various arm movements explore scapular protraction and retraction, and intensify the stretch in the front of the body through bending the elbow overhead. The arm sweeps in *trikonasana* (#8) and *jathara parivrtti* (#12) incorporate external rotation. *Garudasana* (#10) tests balance and range of motion in protraction through a bind.

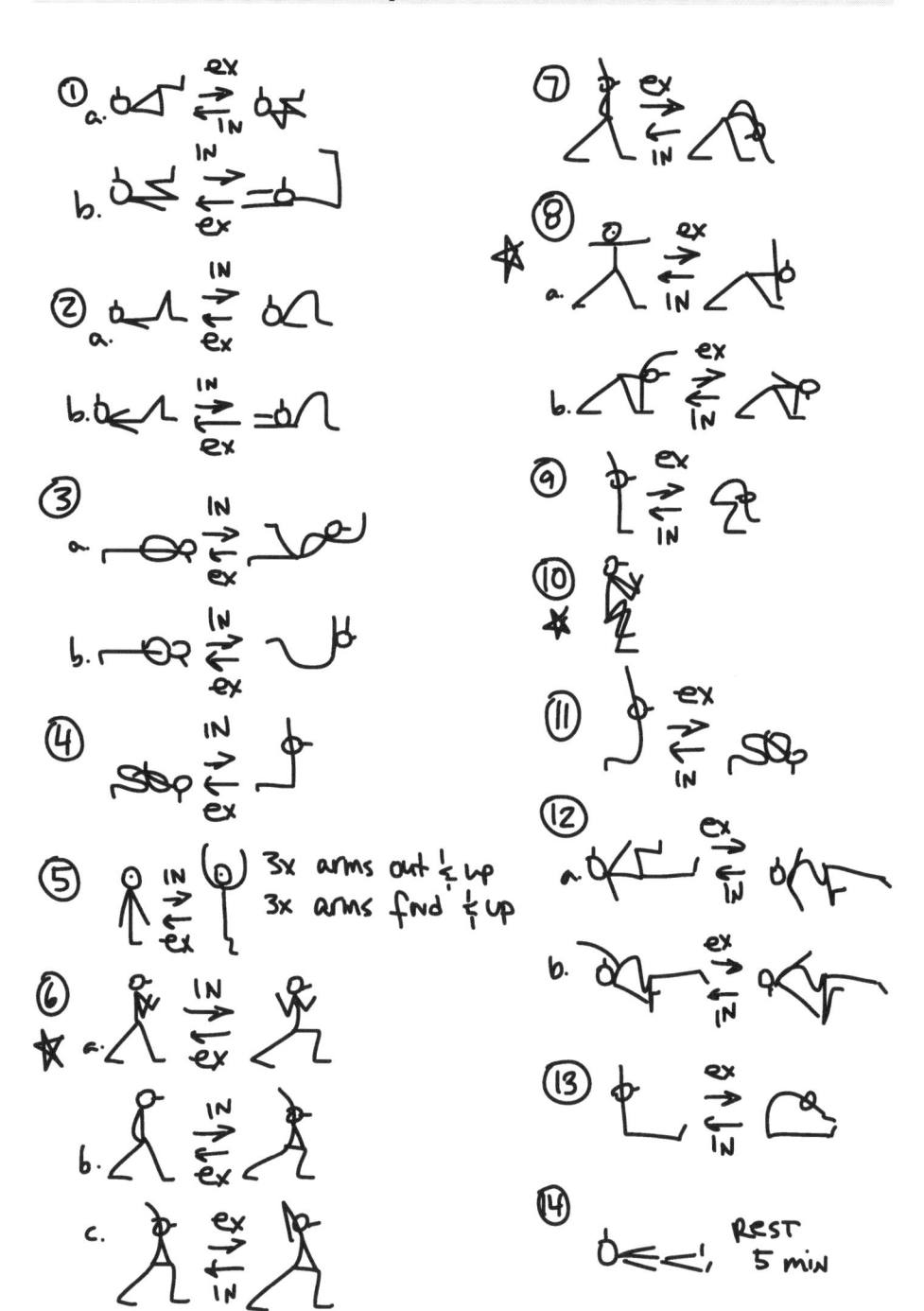

Explore a Joint

8: Potpourri Practice

A potpourri yoga sequence includes a little of everything. Since the scope of a potpourri practice is very broad, use the context of the practice to give it direction. Use the The Magical Worksheet to identify key information that will help you choose postures.

I created this sample sequence for a morning class at a community center with a mixed group of students who prefer an easygoing practice. The core postures are *salabhasana*, *trikonasana*, and *sukhasana parivrtti*. These core postures encompass multiple planes (prone, standing, and seated) as well as different directions of movement (backbend, lateral bend, twist).

Because it is a morning practice, I begin with practitioners lying down to ease gently into movement, where *salabhasana* (#4) the first core posture is introduced. For students who might be uncomfortable in or unable to use kneeling transitions, I've included adaptations using a chair. Then, *trikonasana* (#10) is included at the end of the series of standing postures, and finally *sukhasana parivrtti* (#13) is towards the end of the practice before some final relaxation.

Note how the core postures are spread out throughout the practice. This order is necessary because they are all in different directions and planes and desirable to create a balanced, varied practice.

Potpourri Practice Worksheet

Class: __AM all levels class__   Yoga Sequence Worksheet   Date/Time: __Mon 3/25__

1. **What is the intention?**
   Potpourri practice to start the day

2. **What are the core postures?**
   Prone backbends, standing postures, seated postures

3. **What's the context?**
   Morning practice at a community center

4. **Student demographics & level of experience**
   Wide variety of ages, all have yoga experience

5. **Time of day**
   9:30 AM

6. **Location/other notes**
   Community center, 75 minute class

7. **What do your students WANT?**
   Easygoing practice, self care

8. **What are the potential risks and things to avoid?**
   Avoid complex postures with binds

9. **What else might you take into consideration?**
   No props except chairs

Intention	Context	Time of Day
AM potpourri	Community class	9:30 AM
Core Pose/Seq	Core Pose/Seq	Core Pose/Seq

AM All Levels Potpourri Practice

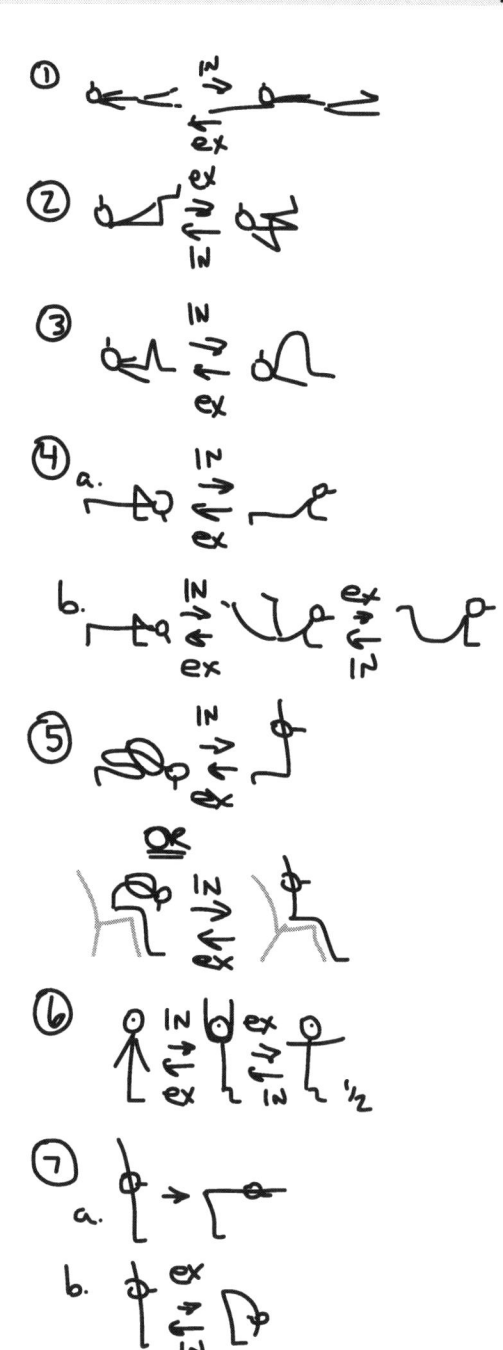

Same Sequence, Different Contexts

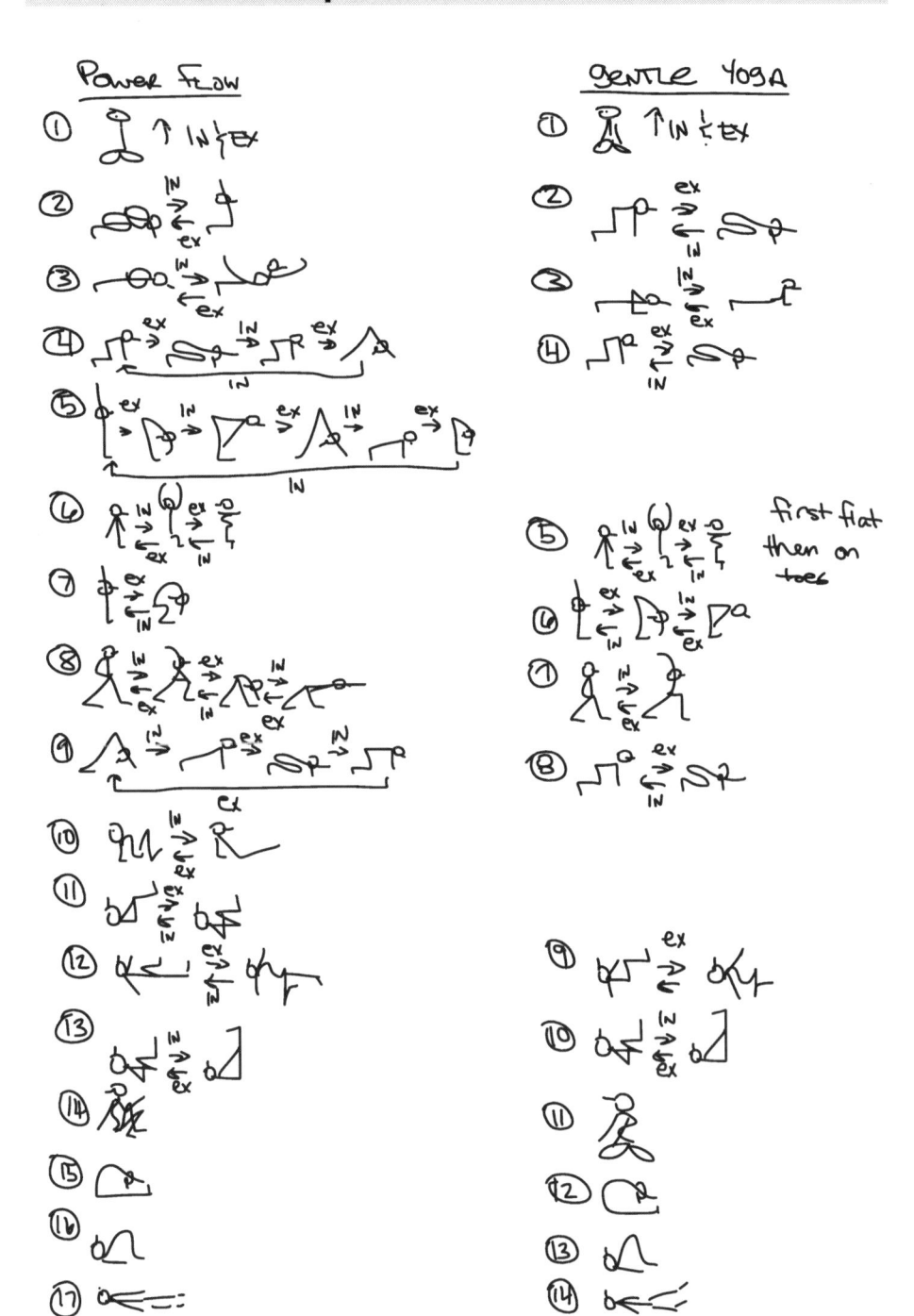

Once you have an understanding of the applications of postures, what makes something simple versus complex, and how context impacts your choice of postures, you can take one idea for a practice and adapt it for various contexts. This approach is particularly useful if you teach multiple classes a week at different locations or to different experience levels.

The following pair of sample sequences demonstrates a potpourri practice that has a little emphasis on twists in two different contexts: a therapeutic power flow class (PF) and a gentle yoga class (GY). Both sequences begin with kneeling forward bends and prone backbends. The gentle yoga practice uses more support with the hands in kneeling and prone positions and revisits *cakravakasana* (GY #4) instead of a variation of sun salutations (PF #4, #5). Likewise, the series of standing postures is more complex and lengthy in the power flow practice, and it is followed by a twisting variation of *navasana* (#10), which is omitted completely in the gentle practice.

Both practices proceed to a supine twist and seated twist, where again the gentle practice uses simpler variations. I've kept the finishing postures, *paschimatanasana* (PF #15, GY #12) and *dwi pada pittham* (PF #16, GY #13) the same.

You can adapt any sequence to any context to influence energetic effects based on time of day, to suit practitioners' experience levels, to account for limitations on time, props available, or otherwise to suit individual needs.

Same Sequence, Different Contexts

Conclusion

Yoga is a profound, multidimensional practice and the scope of this book is the fundamentals sequencing yoga postures. I hope that the principles and tools in this book have inspired you to look at yoga sequences with an analytical eye and approach creating yoga sequences with a newfound sense of purpose. Remember that the heart of yoga teaching is about adapting for the individual. These worksheets, sample sequences, and concepts are adaptable to meet your own needs, so feel free to modify the worksheets or use them as inspiration to make your own practice templates.

For more in-depth study of inner practices of *pranayama*, meditation, and philosophy, including how to craft integrated practices that incorporate all of these elements, I recommend seeking out a Viniyoga therapist in your area at viniyoga.com. I have also included some recommendations for further reading at the end of this book.

This material in this book is also available as an online course, along with my *How to Draw Yoga Stick Figures* video. You can find additional resources for yoga teachers and practitioners at *yogawithflissy.com*.

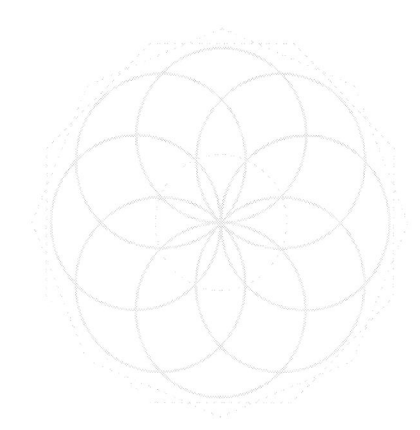

Appendix

Blank Worksheets

Download PDF versions of the following worksheets at:

www.yogawithflissy.com/ysspdfs/pdfworksheets

Class_____ **Yoga Sequence Worksheet** Date/Time:_____

1. What is the intention?

2. What are the core postures?

3. What's the context?

4. Student demographics & level of experience

5. Time of day

6. Location/other notes

7. What do your students WANT?

8. What are the potential risks and things to avoid?

9. What else might you take into consideration?

Intention	Context	Time of Day
Core Pose/Seq	Core Pose/Seq	Core Pose/Seq

Postures	

Class_____   # Yoga Sequence Outline   Date/Time:_____

Intention	Context	Time of Day	Core Pose	Core Pose	Core Pose

Sequence

1. Centering

2. Opening Sequence (joint mobilization)

3. Spine (general warm up, prone backbends, sun salutation A)

4. Hips & Legs (more warmth, sun salutation B, standing postures)

5. Featured Topic (teach a thing!)

6. Seated & Supine (flexibility)

7. Finishing Sequence (compensation and prep for relaxation)

8. Relaxation & Meditation (rest and integration)

Yoga Court Checklist

Sequencing Principles

- ☐ Start with a (simple!) intention
- ☐ Apply general fitness rules
- ☐ Be aware of planes
- ☐ Use proper preparation and compensation
- ☐ Move from simple to complex
- ☐ Consider risks vs. benefits

Yoga Court Questions

- ☐ Do the sequence and included postures reflect the overall intention?
- ☐ Is there appropriate transition between planes?
- ☐ Is there use of forward bends to transition between directions of movement?
- ☐ Does this sequence fit the context in which you'll teach it?
- ☐ Is the sequence efficient and elegant?

Notes:

Further Reading

Bryant, Cedric X. and Daniel J. Green, eds. *ACE Essentials of Exercise Science for Fitness Professionals.* American Council on Exercise, 2017.

Desikachar, T. K. V. *The Heart of Yoga: Developing a Personal Practice.* Inner Traditions International, 1995.

Kaminoff, Leslie. *Yoga Anatomy.* Human Kinetics, 2007.

Kraftsow, Gary. *Yoga for Transformation: Ancient Teachings and Practices for Healing the Body, Mind, and Heart.* Penguin Group, 2002.

Kraftsow, Gary. *Yoga for Wellness: Healing with the Timeless Teachings of Viniyoga.* Penguin Books, 1999.

Schiffmann, Erich. *Yoga: The Spirit and Practice of Moving into Stillness.* Pocket Books, 1996.

Made in the USA
Columbia, SC
03 July 2025